# Anal and rectal diseases explained

## Remedica Explained series

ISSN 1472-4138

*Also available*
Cardiology explained
Interventional radiology explained

*Forthcoming*
Common spinal disorders explained
Nuclear medicine explained



Published by the Remedica Group
Remedica Publishing, 32–38 Osnaburgh Street, London, NW1 3ND, UK
Remedica Inc, Tri-State International Center, Building 25, Suite 150,
Lincolnshire, IL 60069, USA

Email: books@remedica.com
www.remedica.com

Publisher: Andrew Ward
In-house editor: Tamsin White



ISBN 1 901346 67 6
British Library Cataloguing in-Publication Data
A catalogue record for this book is available from the British Library

# Anal and rectal diseases explained

Eli D Ehrenpreis, MD

Assistant Professor of Medicine
Rush Presbyterian St. Luke's Medical Center
Adult Care Specialists
1538 N Arlington Heights Rd
Arlington Heights,
Illinois 60004
USA

# Acknowledgements

I would like to thank the following people for their assistance with this book:

Avrum Epstein, MD, for assistance with radiographic images.

Alessandro Fichera, MD, for manuscript review and additions from a surgical perspective.

Arunas Gasparitus, MD, for providing many interesting and unusual radiographs for the book.

Charles Dye, MD, for providing endoscopic ultrasound images.

Sunanda V Kane, MD, for providing endoscopic photos for the Crohn's disease section.

Andrew Ward for encouraging me to write the book and providing publication support.

Tamsin White for editorial assistance.

# Foreword

This book gives a clear and detailed overview of some of the different anorectal and colonic pathologies. Although some of these conditions are very common in our patient population, our knowledge and our experience in managing these conditions is sometimes lacking. The aim of this book is to provide clinicians with a tool for rapid consultation and a source of information in order to properly answer the patient's questions. Each section clearly describes the condition with up-to-date management guidelines and some very precious clinical pearls.

Each topic is outlined in a multidisciplinary fashion with the medical, surgical, and pathological aspects clearly detailed in each section. Such a succinct overview has long been needed. The format is very clear and certainly this will be a book to have on a ward, in the doctor's office, or on the shelves at home.

Alessandro Fichera, MD
Assistant Professor of Surgery
University of Chicago
Chicago, Illinois

# Contents

# Chapter 1

# General information

# Chapter 1.1

# Anal and rectal anatomy

## Anal canal

The anal canal is the terminal portion of the gastrointestinal tract. It is the short tubular segment, distal to the rectum, which is lined internally by squamous and transitional epithelium. The anal canal begins where the distal rectum penetrates the muscular floor of the pelvic cavity. It is surrounded by the anal sphincter muscle.

## Rectum

The rectum is the distal portion of the large intestine. It is defined as the region lying between the sigmoid colon and the anal canal, and is approximately

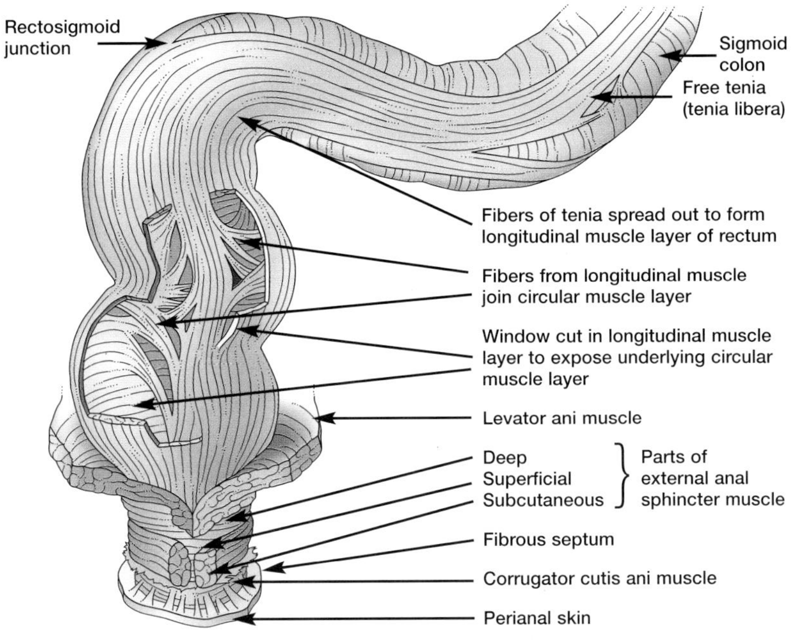


**Figure 1.** Rectal muscular anatomy.

12–15 cm in length. The lower third of the rectum is distal to the peritoneal reflection. Unlike in the rest of the colon, longitudinal muscle fibers in the rectum do not form discrete lengthwise bands (teniae) but, instead, surround the entire rectum (see **Figure 1**). The dentate line marks the distal portion of the rectum and separates it from the anal canal (see **Figure 2**). It also separates two types of epithelia, the simple columnar epithelium of the rectum and the stratified epithelium of the anal canal (anoderm). The dentate line has multiple folds called the columns of Morgagni. The anal crypts and glands are located at the base of the columns of Morgagni. These glands may be the site of perianal abscess and fistula formation. The rectum has three folds, called the valves of Houston.

## Musculature

### Internal anal sphincter

The internal anal sphincter is a thick ring of fibers from the circular smooth muscle of the colon at the proximal portion of the anal canal (see **Figure 3**).

### External anal sphincter

The external anal sphincter surrounds the anal canal at the pelvic diaphragm, distal to the anal orifice (see **Figure 3**). The external anal sphincter is a ring of skeletal muscle, which extends superiorly to the puborectalis, an important constituent of the levator ani, the main muscle of the pelvic floor. Posteriorly, the external anal sphincter has attachments to the coccyx and, anteriorly, to the perineal body. The puborectalis muscle attaches anteriorly to the pubic bone and envelops the lower rectum posteriorly, forming a sling. The puborectalis muscle is responsible for the anorectal angle (see **Section 1.2: The normal process of defecation**).

## Innervation

### Internal anal sphincter

Extrinsic autonomic fibers of both the sympathetic and parasympathetic nervous systems innervate the internal anal sphincter.

### External anal sphincter

The pudendal nerve (sacral nerve roots S3 and S4) innervates the external anal sphincter, the levator ani, and the puborectalis muscles (see **Figure 4**).

### Rectum

The rectum is innervated by the sympathetic nervous system via the pelvic plexus (L1, L2, and L3), and the parasympathetic nervous system via the nervi erigentes (S2, S3, and S4).

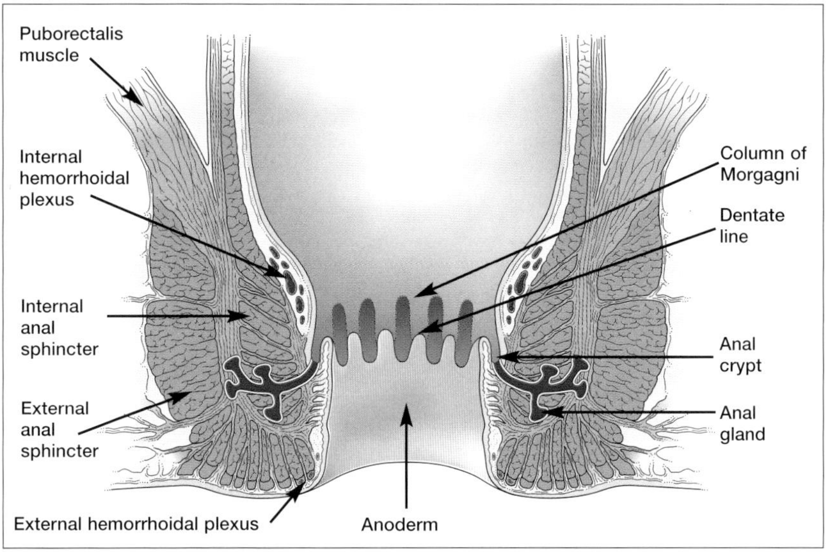


**Figure 2.** Anatomy of the anal region.

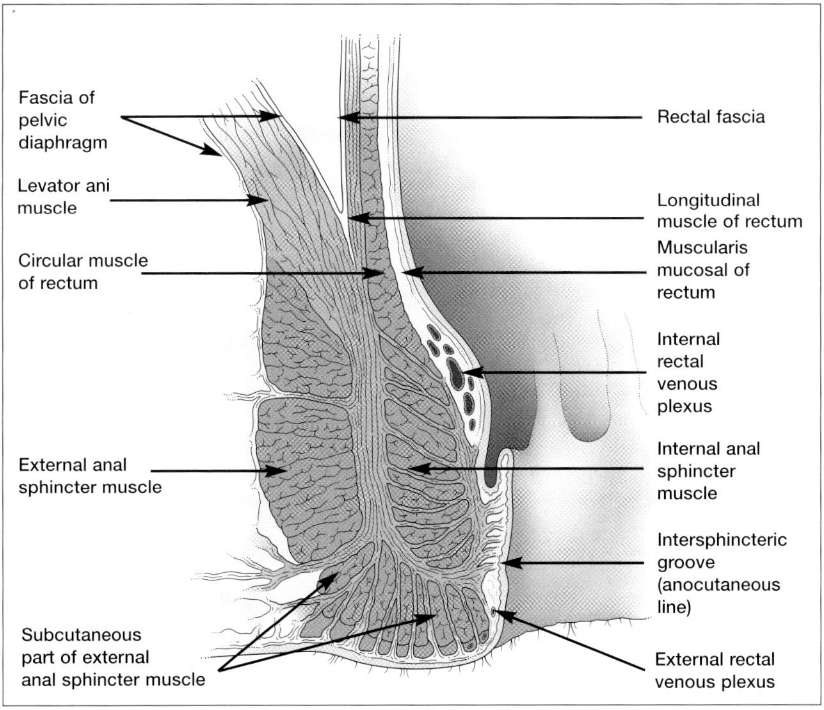


**Figure 3.** Anal muscular anatomy.

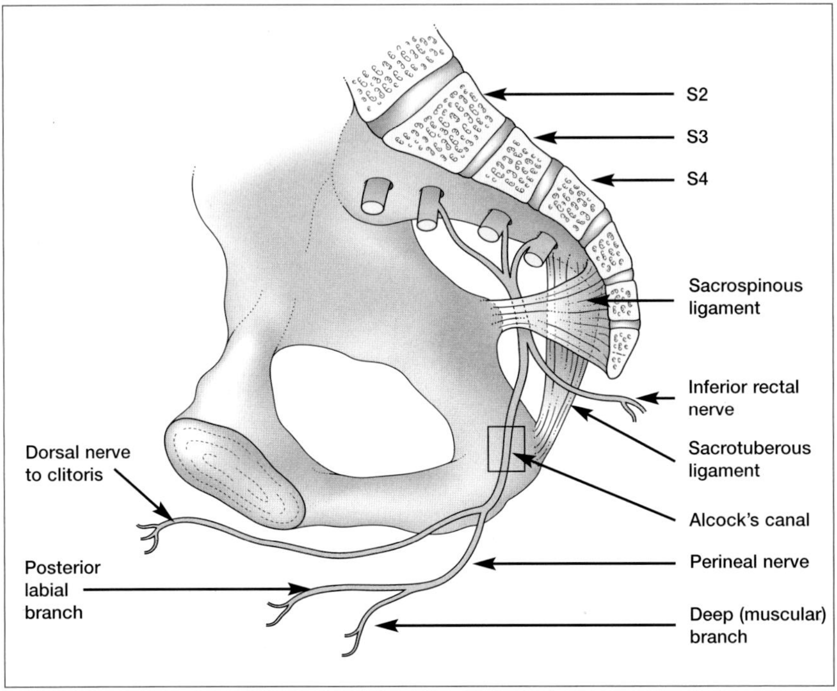


**Figure 4.** The branches of the pudendal nerve.

# Vascular supply

## Anal

### *Arterial*

The superior, middle, and inferior rectal arteries supply blood to the anus.

### *Venous*

Internal hemorrhoidal plexus: connects to the superior rectal veins, which drain into the inferior mesenteric vein, which connects to the portal venous system.

External hemorrhoidal plexus: connects to the middle rectal veins and pudendal veins, which drain into the internal iliac vein, which connects to the inferior vena cava.

## Rectal

### *Arterial*

Arterial supply to the rectum occurs via the superior rectal, middle rectal, and inferior rectal arteries (see **Figure 5**). The superior rectal artery is a branch of the inferior mesenteric artery. The middle rectal artery originates from the internal iliac

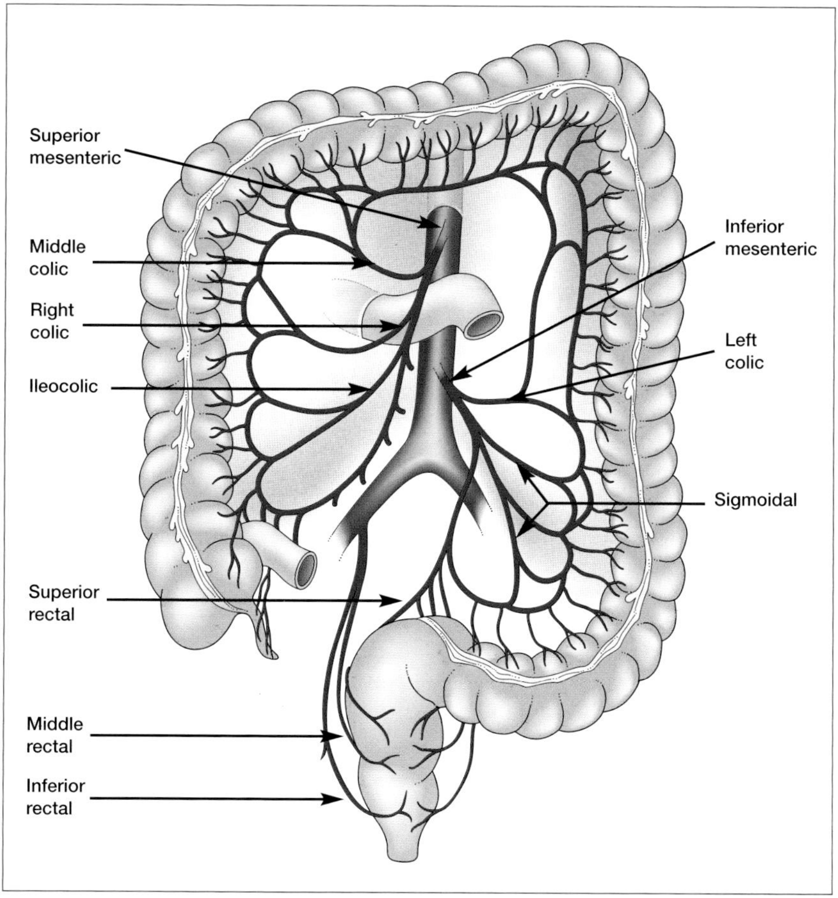


**Figure 5.** The arterial supply to the colon originates from the superior and inferior mesenteric arteries.

or the pudendal artery, and the inferior rectal artery originates from the internal iliac artery. The majority of the blood supply is from the superior and inferior rectal arteries.

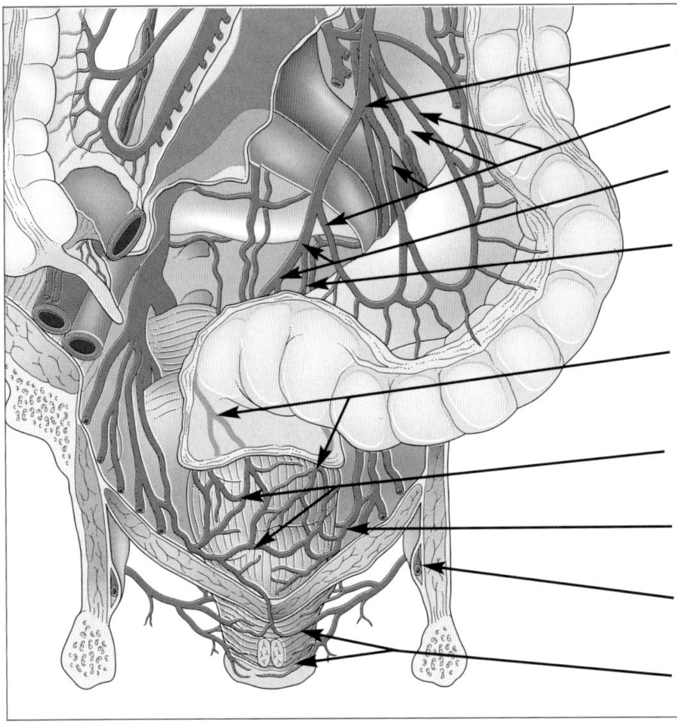

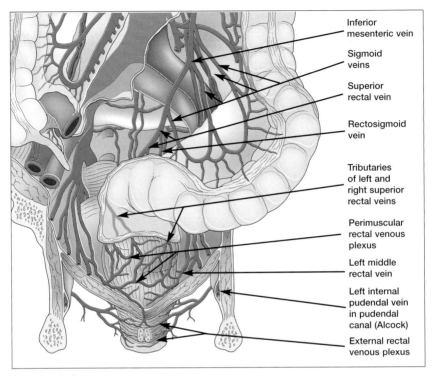

**Figure 6.** Rectal venous anatomy.

### *Venous*

Venous drainage of the majority of the rectum occurs via the middle rectal vein, which connects to the inferior vena cava, and the superior rectal vein, which connects to the portal vein (see **Figure 6**).

# Chapter 1.2

# The normal process of defecation

The neuromuscular anatomy of the anus and rectum is "designed" to preserve fecal continence and to facilitate defecation: withholding stool until it is appropriate to defecate and propelling stool at the time of defecation.

The puborectalis muscle remains tonically contracted at rest to form the anorectal angle, a sharp angulation (normally approximately 90°), which blocks stool from exiting out of the rectum (see **Figures 1** and **2**). The anal sphincters further function to provide a barrier for the passage of air, fluid, or solid stool to exit out of the anal canal.

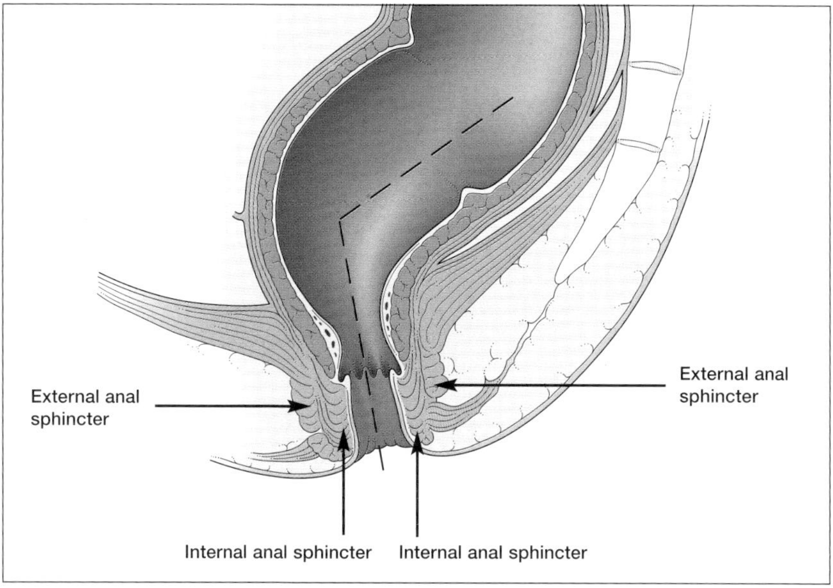


**Figure 1.** The pull of the puborectalis anteriorly towards the pubis muscle contributes to the angulation between the rectum and anal canal termed the anorectal angle (dashed line).

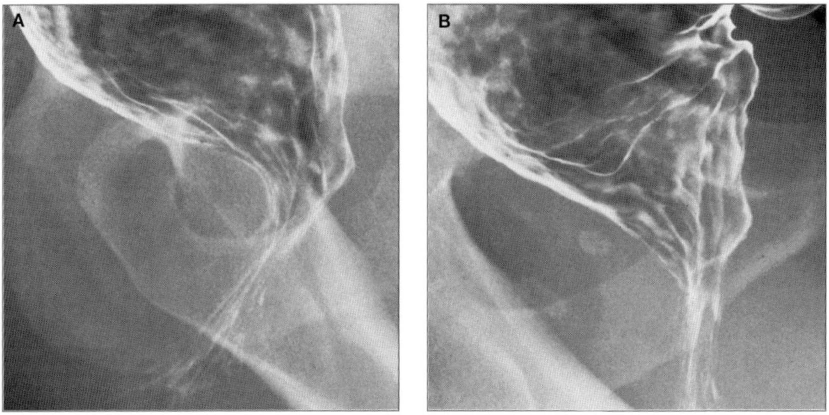


**Figure 2.** Normal dynamic proctogram (**A**) at rest and (**B**) straining demonstrating straightening of the anorectal angle

When stool enters the rectum (which is a highly compliant organ), it distends and the internal anal sphincter (which is normally contracted) relaxes while the external anal sphincter remains closed. This process is called the rectoanal inhibitory reflex and is defective in Hirschsprung's disease. When stool is present in the rectum but defecation is not to be initiated, the puborectalis muscle and external anal sphincter remain contracted. At the appropriate time for defecation, the puborectalis muscle relaxes and the anorectal angle increases, contraction of the diaphragm and abdominal muscles increases interabdominal pressure, relaxation of the external anal sphincter occurs, and feces are passed in conjunction with contraction of the rectum (see **Figure 3**). Increased contraction of the puborectalis muscle and external anal sphincter will occur when there is sensation of stool within the anal canal and voluntary defecation has not been initiated.

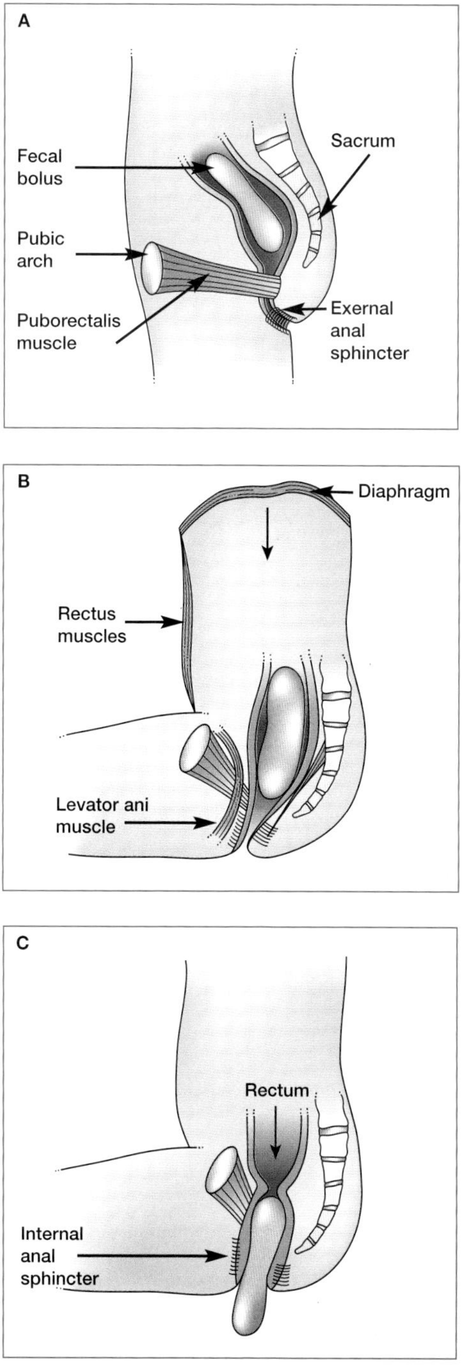


**Figure 3.** The process of defecation. **(A)** Puborectalis and external sphincter are contracted at rest. **(B)** With entry of stool into the rectum, the puborectalis and anal sphincters relax; the levator ani, rectus muscles, and diaphragm contract. **(C)** With defecation, the external anal sphincter relaxes; there is a rectal contraction.

# Chapter 2

# Diagnostic procedures

# Chapter 2.1

# Anorectal manometry

## Description of procedure

Anorectal manometry is widely used to diagnose abnormalities of anorectal function. This test employs a pressure-sensitive catheter connected to a transducer. The catheter device is inserted into the anus and anal pressure is measured throughout the length of the anal canal. The transducer translates the mechanical pressures into an electrical signal, which is converted to a computerized readout and used to interpret the data obtained.

## Indications

Chronic constipation, fecal incontinence, documentation of the presence or absence of rectoanal inhibitory reflex (RAIR) for the diagnosis of Hirschsprung's disease (see **Figure 1**), and preoperative use prior to ileoanal pouch or colorectal anastomosis. Anorectal manometry can also be used as an adjunctive tool for performance of anorectal biofeedback.

## Complementary procedures

Dynamic proctography, anorectal electromyography (EMG) and pudendal nerve terminal motor latency study (PNTML), flexible sigmoidoscopy, full-thickness biopsy of the rectum (for diagnosis of Hirschsprung's disease), and anorectal ultrasound.

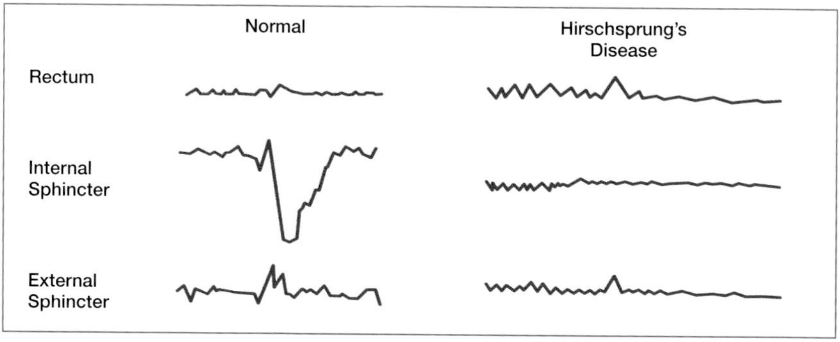


**Figure 1.** The rectoanal inhibitory reflex (RAIR) demonstrated in a normal subject and absent in a patient with Hirschsprung's disease.

## Contraindications

Anal obstruction.

## Relative contraindications

Severe anal pain and anal stricture.

## Preparation of patient

The patient should receive one or two sodium phosphate enemas several hours prior to examination. You should also talk with them prior to the procedure to answer any concerns they may have so that they are relaxed and cooperative when the procedure begins.

## How the procedure is performed

The patient is placed in a left lateral position with flexion of the knees and hips, and proper draping for adequate modesty. Pressure-sensitive catheters (balloon system, water perfusion system, or solid-state microtransducer system) are gently placed in the anal canal following calibration of the manometer. The pressure is measured through eight channels placed around the catheter, each 1 cm apart and extending 5 cm from the distal portion of the catheter. The pressure in each channel is generally measured with a "pull-through technique" (the probe is placed in the rectum and gradually withdrawn) (see **Figure 2**).

The pressure readings obtained provide a longitudinal pressure profile of the anal sphincter. The parameters measured are discussed below.

### High-pressure zone

The high-pressure zone (HPZ) is usually present 1–1.5 cm proximal to the anal verge. This is a portion of the anal canal where pressures are greater than 50% above the average pressures within the remainder of the anal canal

### Resting pressure

Resting pressure is measured at the HPZ. The average value is 65–85 mm Hg.

### Squeeze pressure

The patient performs a squeezing maneuver of the anus following an explanation by the performing technician. These pressures are usually 50%–100% higher than the average resting pressure.

### Push pressure

The patient is instructed to perform the push maneuver, mimicking an attempt to defecate. The measured pressure tracings are then viewed to determine whether a normal decrease in anal pressure occurs.

### RAIR

Following the above maneuvers, a latex balloon is placed over the manometry catheter, which is then repositioned 2 cm from the anal verge. Small volumes of air are introduced into the balloon (typically beginning with 40 mL). Baseline resting anal pressures are measured to determine whether resting pressures decrease following inflation of the balloon. This decrease in sphincter pressure is called "RAIR". If no reflex is detected, the balloon is deflated and reinflated at a higher volume, such as 60 mL. Volumes of up to 180 mL may be required to document the presence of RAIR.

### Detection of rectal sensation

The aforementioned balloon inflation using air or water at room temperature is performed and utilized to determine: 1) the volume required to elicit an initial sensation; 2) the volume required to produce a sensation of urgency; and 3) the maximum tolerable volume. Volumes of up to 300 mL may be utilized to determine rectal volume sensation.

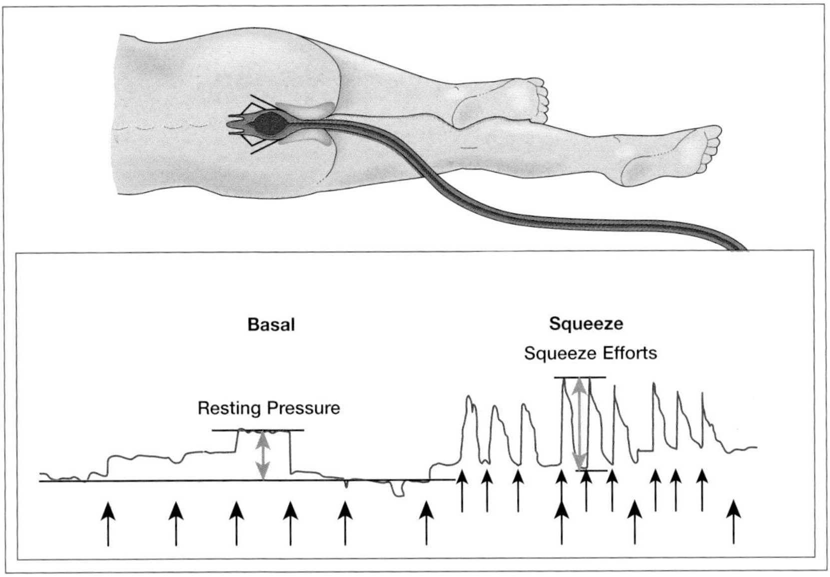


**Figure 2.** Demonstration of the high-pressure zone and resting and squeeze pressures using a pull-through technique.

Pressure measurements may be used to map the symmetry of the anal sphincter. The presence of marked anal asymmetry is seen with sphincter damage or other abnormalities.

Changes in pressure with balloon inflation at different volumes may be used to determine rectal compliance. These studies are generally used for research purposes. Rectal compliance measurements have been used to show, for example, that some patients with irritable bowel syndrome have decreased rectal compliance, enhancing the sense of urgency experienced in the condition.

## Typical abnormal findings

The most common abnormal findings on anorectal manometry and the possible causes of these abnormalities are shown in **Table 1**.

## Complications

None.

## Additional comments

Biofeedback techniques have been successfully utilized in conjunction with anorectal manometry to assist with retraining of the anal sphincter in patients with fecal incontinence and spastic anorectal disorders.

| Finding | Cause |
|---|---|
| Elevated resting pressure | Anal sphincter spasm (anismus), nonrelaxing puborectalis syndrome, hemorrhoids, or anal fissure |
| Decreased resting and squeeze pressures | Anal injury secondary to trauma, anal surgery or obstetric injury, neurologic diseases, or anorectal prolapse |
| Absence of the fall in resting anal pressure with push maneuver | Anismus or nonrelaxing puborectalis syndrome |
| Absence of RAIR | Hirschsprung's disease or megacolon/megarectum |
| Lowered threshold of rectal sensation | Irritable bowel syndrome or post-gastroenteritis hypersensitivity |
| Decreased rectal sensation | Altered sensorium, central nervous system disease, neurologic disorders, or megacolon/megarectum |
| Decreased rectal compliance | Colitis, radiation proctopathy, or irritable bowel syndrome |

**Table 1.** Common abnormal findings on anorectal manometry and their possible causes. RAIR: rectoanal inhibitory reflex.

# Chapter 2.2

# Anoscopy and proctoscopy

## Description of procedure

Anoscopy (endoscopic examination of anal mucosa and lower rectum) and proctoscopy (endoscopic examination of entire rectum) involve the placement of a rigid plastic or metal instrument (anoscope/proctoscope – see **Figure 1**) into the anal canal. The proctoscope has either an internal or external light source.

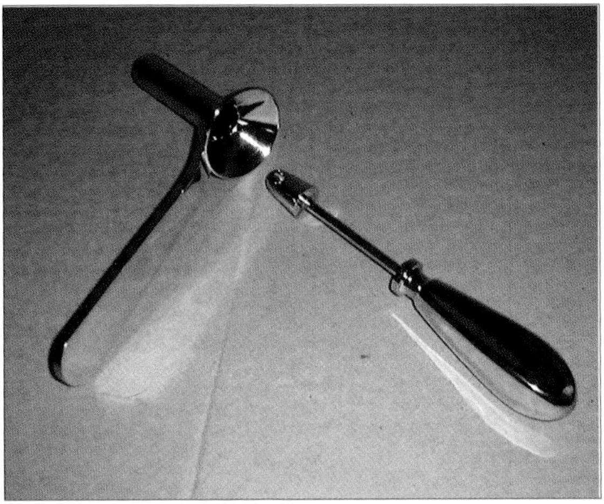

**Figure 1.** A Naunton Morgan proctoscope (image courtesy of B & H Surgical Instrument Makers, London, UK).

## Indications

Anal pain, discharge, rectal bleeding, internal or external hemorrhoids, pruritus ani, palpable mass on digital rectal examination, or anal condyloma.

## Complementary procedures

Flexible sigmoidoscopy and colonoscopy.

## Contraindications

Acute myocardial infarction (due to the potential of inducing a vagal response) and a patient who is unable/unwilling to cooperate with the procedure.

## Relative contraindications

Suspected acute abdomen, debilitated patient, or anal stenosis.

## Preparation of patient

Patient reassurance is mandatory. Generally, no preparation is required for the procedure, although an enema may be used if necessary.

## How the procedure is performed

The patient is placed in a left lateral position. A local anesthetic may be applied to the anal region. A digital examination is performed after lubrication of the gloved finger. The anoscope or proctoscope is lubricated and placed gently into the anus. This is advanced slowly following relaxation of the anal sphincter. Sometimes, gentle rotation of the device eases insertion. After full advancement of the scope, the inner obturator is removed. Suctioning may be performed to clear the view and a light source is utilized to obtain good visualization. The scope is gently withdrawn for evaluation and the walls of the anus and rectum are viewed. Biopsies and suctioning of fecal material for culture and microscopy may be performed.

## Typical abnormal findings

Anal or rectal lesions such as hemorrhoids or neoplasms. Biopsies of lesions may be obtained, and suctioned material collected for culture and microscopic evaluation. The collected material is useful for diagnosing sexually transmitted diseases of the anus and rectum.

## Complications

Patient discomfort and/or embarrassment are common. Uncommon complications include tearing of the anoderm or postbiopsy bleeding.

## Additional comments

Anoscopy and proctoscopy have been replaced by flexible sigmoidoscopy in many clinical practices.

# Chapter 2.3

# Barium enema

## Description of procedure

A barium enema is a radiographic examination of the colon (see **Figure 1**). It is performed using either a single column of barium sulfate instilled into the colon, or a barium instillation combined with air to perform an air–contrast study.

## Indications

Evaluation of symptoms suggestive of colonic disease, such as constipation, rectal bleeding, irritable bowel syndrome, and unexplained diarrhea. Complete evaluation of the colon for colorectal cancer screening or surveillance when colonoscopy is contraindicated or cannot be safely or adequately performed.

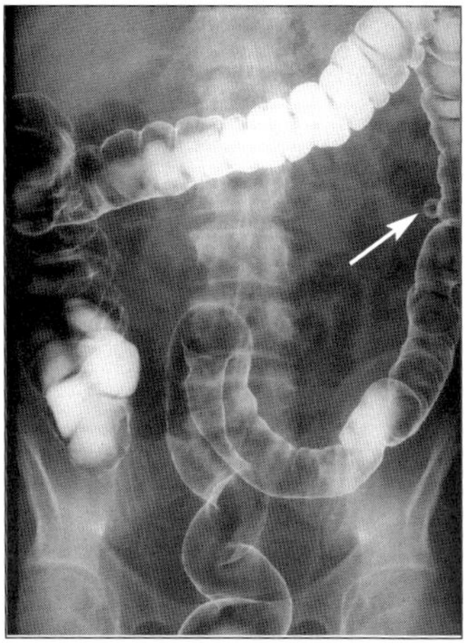

**Figure 1a.** Normal view of the colon on barium enema examination. A single diverticulum is noted in the descending colon (arrow).

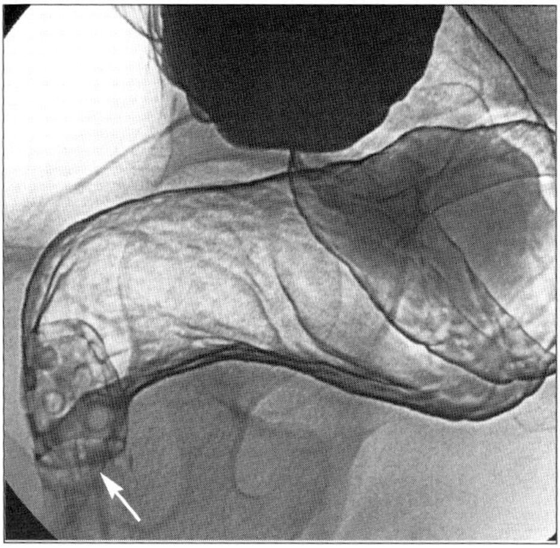

**Figure 1b.** Normal view of the rectum on barium enema. Enema tip is present (arrow).

## Complementary procedures

Colonoscopy, anorectal manometry, anorectal electromyography (EMG), defecography, abdominal and pelvic computed tomography (CT) scan, stool culture, stool microscopy, stool for *Clostridium difficile* toxin testing, fecal fat testing, and electrolyte examination.

## Contraindications

Prior allergic reaction to barium, imperforate anus, bowel obstruction, or tight stricture of the colon.

## Relative contraindications

Inability to prepare a patient, a patient who is unwilling or unable to cooperate with the procedure, or a colonic stricture.

## Preparation of patient

This usually takes place over 2 days. On day 1, patients begin a low residue diet with encouragement of liquid intake. On day 2, patients initiate a clear liquid diet. This is complemented by administration of laxatives, enemas, and/or suppositories. In our practice, patients are encouraged to drink one 8 oz bottle of magnesium citrate at 12:00 (midday) on day 2. This is followed by two bisacodyl tablets at 16:00 and 20:00. Clear liquids are encouraged until 22:00, after which no further intake of food or liquids is allowed. At 06:00 on the day of the study, the patient self-administers one bisacodyl suppository.

## How the procedure is performed

The technician places a catheter into the rectum and barium is injected to fill the colon. Intravenous glucagon is often administered to assist with distribution of the barium. Barium placed into the colon provides contrast material to outline colonic lesions and makes them visible on x-ray films. Fluoroscopy is used (with the patient in a supine position) to visualize the posterior portions of the colon, and with the patient in a prone position to evaluate the anterior colonic walls. Patients are turned periodically to coat the entire colon with barium. Subsequently, air is instilled to provide air contrast by spreading the barium into a thin layer along the colonic wall. A balloon is placed and inflated in the rectum to prevent discharge of the barium. During the procedure, fluoroscopy and static x-rays are obtained at various angles to visualize all regions of the colon. After evacuation of the barium, the images of the colon are examined for mucosal abnormalities and anatomic disruptions.

## Typical abnormal findings

Alterations of colonic anatomy such as tortuosity and increased length of the sigmoid colon in chronic constipation or loss of haustration in cases of laxative abuse. The barium enema may reveal causes of constipation, abdominal or pelvic pain, and diarrhea, such as obstructing colonic lesions, severe diverticular disease (see **Figure 2**), ulcerative colitis, and Crohn's disease.

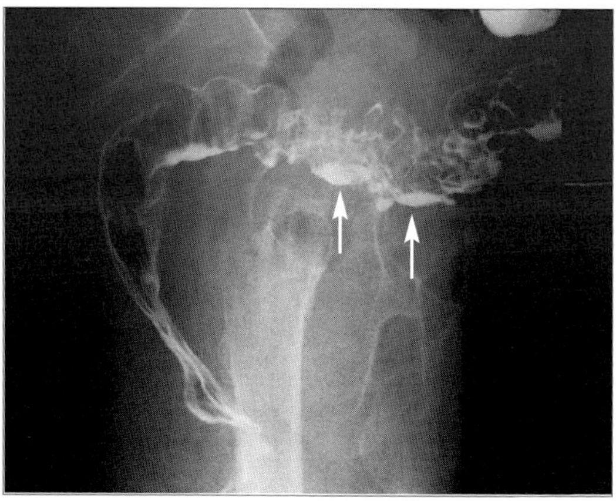

**Figure 2.** Marked sigmoid diverticulosis (arrows) demonstrated on barium enema. The colon is poorly distensible.

## Complications

Barium enemas are usually very well tolerated, although discomfort and embarrassment are common during the procedure. Perforation, dehydration, barium concretion, severe constipation, and obstipation are relatively rare.

## Additional comments

Barium enema examination will miss up to 10% of colorectal cancers and colonic polyps and is therefore not recommended as a first-line procedure for colorectal cancer screening or surveillance. The inflated rectal balloon that is present during the performance of the barium enema limits visualization of the rectum, therefore, a proctoscopy or sigmoidoscopy is required for complete colonic evaluation. Barium enemas may be combined with defecography in a single test for constipation. In our practice, this combined test is used in patients with chronic constipation to rule out anatomic abnormalities and to evaluate for the presence of pelvic floor disorders.

# Chapter 2.4

# Biofeedback therapy

## Description of procedure

Biofeedback therapy is a form of pelvic muscular retraining.

## Indications

Chronic constipation and fecal incontinence.

## Complementary procedures

Kegel exercises, defecography, balloon expulsion testing, testing of rectal sensation, and intrasphincteric botulinum toxin (Botox) injections.

## Contraindications

Imperforate anus.

## Relative contraindications

Inability of the patient to understand or cooperate with the procedure.

## Preparation of patient

Some centers recommend that patients use two Fleet's enemas on the morning of the procedure: others perform the procedure without preparation with Fleet's enemas.

## How the procedure is performed

Anal electromyography (EMG) or anorectal manometry are used to provide biofeedback during pelvic retraining. Exercises are generally performed for 1 hour per week. Initially, patients are educated on the function of the pelvic floor muscles, often with the use of a video demonstration. This increases patient understanding and compliance, and encourages patient participation in the procedure.

Patients are then taught to appreciate the difference in sensation between anal resting, squeezing, and pushing. Measurements of anal pressures and activity during these maneuvers are obtained using anorectal manometry or EMG. Patients perform Kegel exercises and relaxation techniques at home and chart home bowel activities. Follow-up sessions with manometry or EMG measurements are performed. Biofeedback therapists use reinforcement techniques and set specific objective goals (based on manometric or EMG measurements) for resting, pushing, and squeezing maneuvers. Biofeedback therapists may utilize additional techniques during the sessions to assist patients in stress management, proper bathroom goals, and lifestyle modification.

## Results obtained

A number of studies have demonstrated that biofeedback therapy is highly successful for the treatment of pelvic floor-related defecation disorders (84% of patients undergoing the procedure report improvement in their symptoms). This technique is also relatively successful in patients with fecal incontinence.

## Complications

There are no complications *per se*; the technique is usually well tolerated, although mild discomfort may occur.

## Additional comments

Biofeedback therapy has also been utilized for the treatment of other forms of chronic constipation and for irritable bowel syndrome.

# Chapter 2.5

# Colonoscopy

## Description of procedure

A colonoscopy is an endoscopic investigation of the colon using a colonoscope; a flexible device that is 8–12 mm in diameter and 120–230 cm in length (see **Figure 1**). It is inserted into the anal canal and advanced proximally to the cecum (and at times to the terminal ileum) (see **Figure 2**). The colonoscope provides a well-lit, magnified view of the colonic mucosa. It has a suction channel to remove fecal material for analysis and a biopsy port to obtain mucosal specimens for histologic evaluation. Hemostasis of bleeding lesions can be performed through this channel using injection therapy with epinephrine and thermal coagulation therapy.

## Indications

Evaluation of an abnormality seen on barium enema; gastrointestinal bleeding; unexplained iron deficiency anemia; surveillance of patients with a history of colon cancer or colonic polyps; screening of high-risk individuals for colon cancer or colonic polyps; screening of normal individuals for colon cancer or colonic polyps; evaluation of patients with chronic inflammatory bowel disease or unexplained diarrhea; and intraoperative evaluation of colonic lesions.

## Complementary procedures

Small intestine radiography, upper endoscopy, and computed tomography (CT) scan of the abdomen and pelvis.

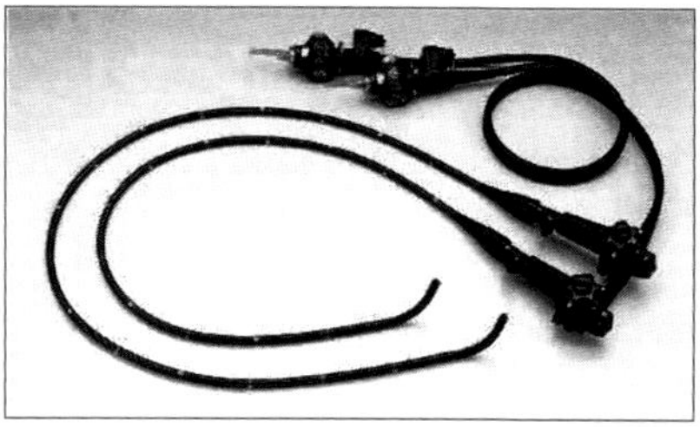

**Figure 1.** A colonoscope (CF240DLI - courtesy of KeyMed Ltd).

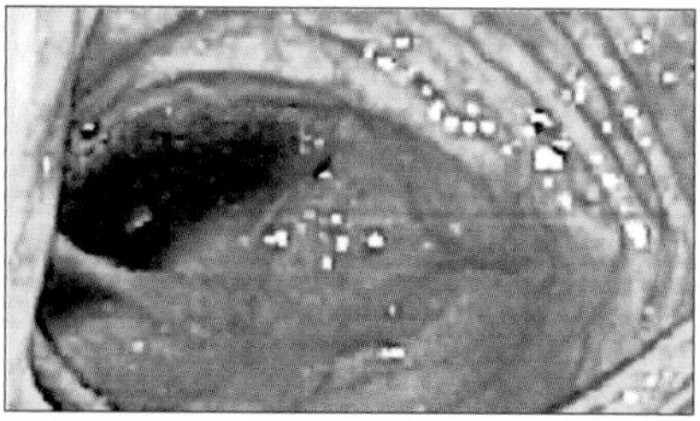

**Figure 2.** The base of the cecum and ileocecal valve demonstrated on colonoscopy.

## Contraindications

Fulminant colitis, acute severe diverticulitis, and suspected gastrointestinal perforation.

## Relative contraindications

Inability to prepare for the procedure (since the colon must be purged for a complete evaluation), inability to obtain consent for the procedure, lack of intravenous access, inability to provide adequate sedation to complete examination, and coagulopathy.

## Preparation of patient

This generally begins the day prior to the procedure. A clear liquid diet is started in the afternoon before the colonoscopy. On the evening before the procedure, the patient should consume 4 L of polyethylene glycol in a balanced electrolyte solution over 2–5 hours. An alternative preparation in younger, healthier patients is two 45-mL doses of oral Fleet's phosphosoda (sodium phosphate 3.3 g/5 mL), one on the evening prior to the procedure and one on the morning of the procedure; each dose should be accompanied by 1.25 L of clear liquids. An oral sodium phosphate preparation in tablet form has recently been introduced.

## How the procedure is performed

The patient is usually placed in a left lateral position. Intravenous sedation (usually combining an opioid such as meperidine and a benzodiazepine such as midazolam or diazepam) is administered. A digital rectal examination is performed. The colonoscope is introduced and advanced to the cecum. External pressure and position changes are often required to allow a safe, full evaluation of the colon. If Crohn's disease is suspected, or a more proximal source of gastrointestinal bleeding is considered, the ileocecal valve is traversed and the colonoscope is introduced into the terminal ileum. After confirmation of the location of the tip of the colonoscope in the cecum, the scope is gradually withdrawn.

Any polyps that are seen on colonoscope withdrawal are removed. Techniques for polyp removal include snaring the polyp with or without electrocautery and performance of a biopsy with associated electrocautery. Multiple biopsies are performed on suspected cancers or lesions that are too large to remove with the colonoscope. If patients are evaluated for unexplained diarrhea, biopsies of the colon (and sometimes the ileum) are obtained in abnormal as well as apparently normal mucosa.

In patients with ulcerative colitis or Crohn's disease who are receiving colonoscopic surveillance, biopsies are obtained from each of the four quadrants every 10 cm for histologic evaluation to rule out dysplasia. Retroflexion of the colonoscope in the distal rectum allows visualization of the proximal anal canal and the dentate line. This is particularly useful when looking for internal hemorrhoids and distal rectal or high anal canal lesions. The retroflexed view is also useful for finding and removing polyps in the distal rectum.

## Typical abnormal findings

Full evaluation of the colonic mucosa is obtained with colonoscopy. Identification and removal of colonic polyps is performed (see **Figures 3–5**). Identification of sources of colonic bleeding (see **Figures 6** and **7**); evaluation of the distal rectum and anal canal for bleeding sources; diagnosis of inflammatory bowel disease; determination of endoscopic and histologic severity of inflammatory bowel disease; surveillance of those carrying the diagnosis of ulcerative colitis or Crohn's disease; and diagnosis of microscopic colitis.

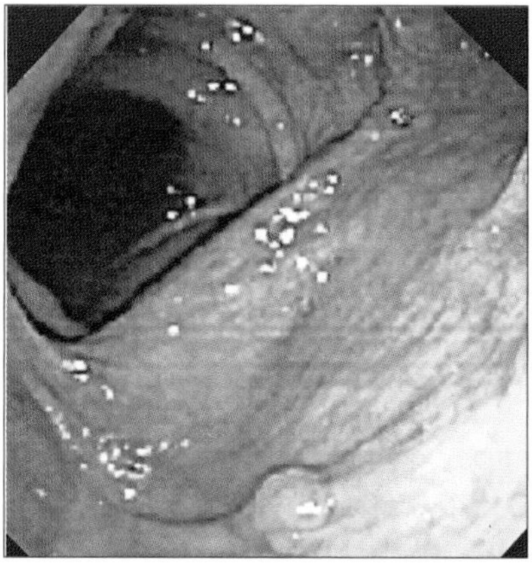

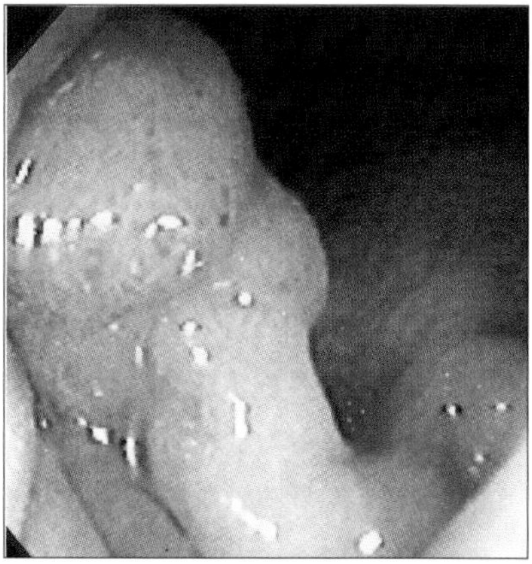

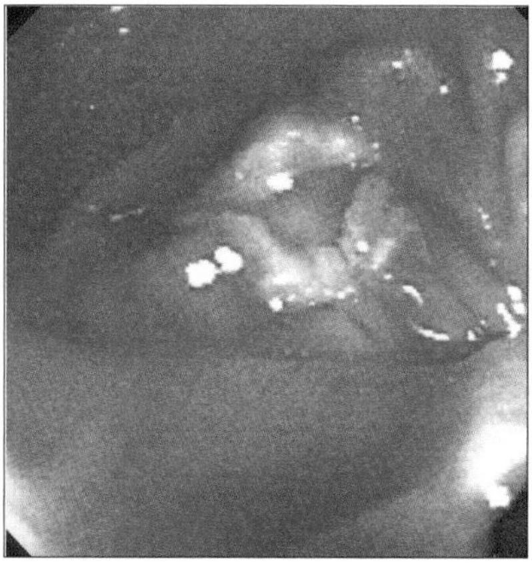

**Figure 3.** A sessile polyp of the ascending colon (top left).

**Figure 4.** A pedunculated polyp in the descending colon (above).

**Figure 5.** Polypectomy site after snare and electrocautery of a polyp (bottom left).

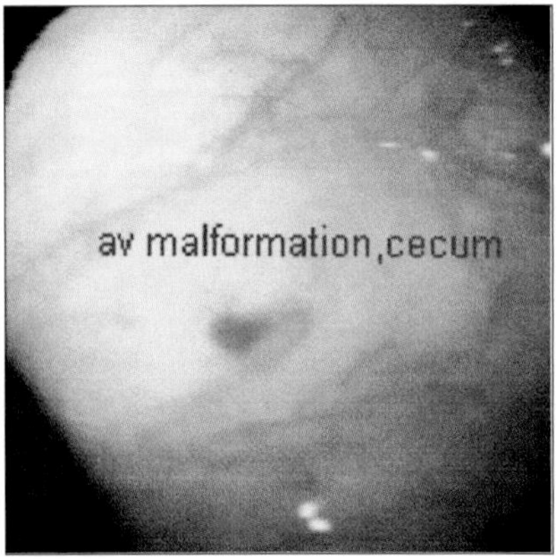


**Figure 6.** Cecal arteriovenous malformation.

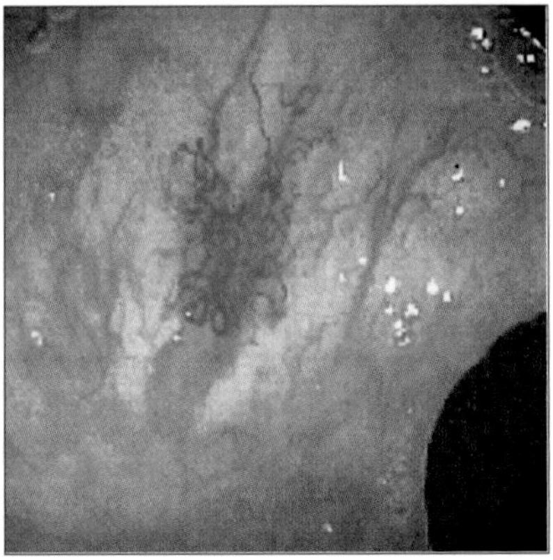

**Figure 7.** Arteriovenous malformation of ascending colon.

## Complications

The perforation rate for colonoscopy is estimated to be between 0.2%–1% (depending on whether a polypectomy has been performed). Postpolypectomy bleeding ranges from 0.4% to 2%. Dehydration and electrolyte abnormalities – including hypernatremia, hyponatremia, hypokalemia, and hypomagnesemia – may occur with sodium phosphate-based colonoscopy preparations. Recently, several cases of severe hyponatremia have been described after polyethylene glycol preparation. Respiratory depression, hypotension, and bradycardia associated with excessive sedation are infrequent. Patients generally experience some discomfort during the procedure.

## Additional comments

New techniques for colon cancer screening, including CT of the colon (virtual colonoscopy) and molecular biology based stool testing, are under investigation.

# Chapter 2.6

# Dynamic proctography

## Description of procedure

A small quantity (about 250 mL) of high viscosity barium is placed in the rectum. Subjects are then seated on a radiolucent commode. Lateral fluoroscopy is performed following identification of the anal canal. The radiologist instructs the patient to hold the barium to allow films to be taken at rest, and to squeeze the anus shut to hold in the barium to obtain "squeeze" films. Finally, the patient is asked to strain and attempt to evacuate the barium. Continuous video fluoroscopy is the preferred method of obtaining data. Static views are also obtained and the anatomic position of the pubococcygeal line is determined. Lateral films are utilized to measure the anorectal angle between the anal canal and the horizontal axis of the rectum (located approximately 2 cm above the ischial tuberosity). This technique can identify changes in the anorectal angle, alteration of anorectal anatomy, and abnormal mobility of the pelvic floor with the aforementioned maneuvers.

## Indications

Constipation, fecal incontinence, identification of rectovaginal fistulas, and evaluation of ileoanal pouch anastomoses.

## Complementary procedures

Barium enema, anorectal electromyography (EMG), anorectal ultrasound, and colonoscopy.

## Contraindications

Allergy to barium, imperforate anus, or tight rectal stricture.

## Relative contraindications

Inability of the patient to cooperate with the procedure.

## Preparation of patient

Most radiologists recommend colonic cleansing using a saline-based cathartic laxative such as magnesium citrate and/or enemas. A few perform the procedure without prior preparation.

## How the procedure is performed

As described above. Analysis of static and dynamic data is required. In normal patients, the anorectal angle is approximately 90° at rest, increasing to >135° with straining and defecation, and decreasing to about 75° with squeeze maneuvers (see **Figures 1** and **2**). The presence of a widened resting anorectal angle can be seen in patients with neurogenic incontinence. Abnormalities such as rectoceles and anorectal intussusception can also be determined during maneuvers.

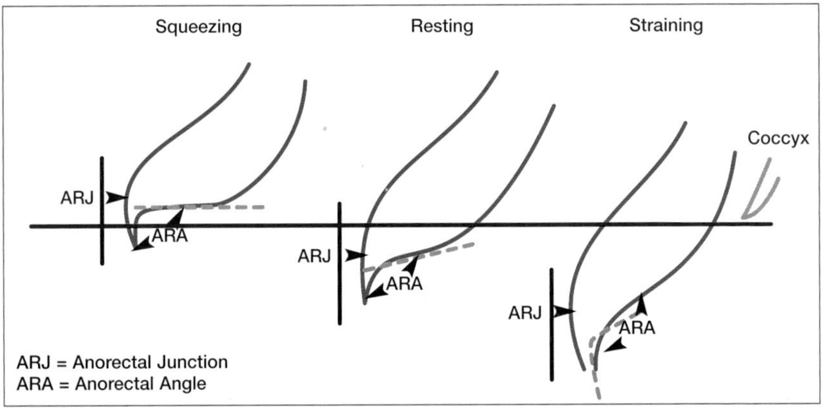


**Figure 1.** Normal changes of the anorectal angle and anal canal seen with maneuvers during dynamic proctography.

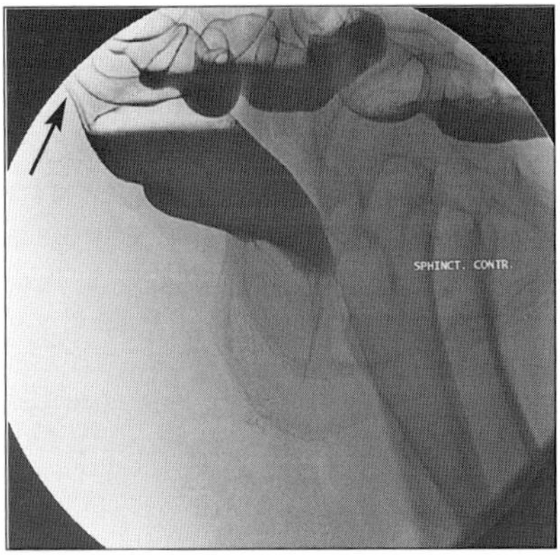


**Figure 2.** Squeeze maneuver on dynamic proctography. Barium does not move into the anal canal due to contraction of the puborectalis muscle (arrow).

## Typical abnormal findings

Dynamic proctography may reveal abnormalities as described above. Alterations in the anorectal angle can be seen, and nonrelaxing puborectalis syndrome or anismus can be diagnosed. Rectocele (see **Figure 3**), abnormal pelvic descent, anorectal intussusception, anovaginal fistula (see **Figure 4**), pubococcygeal tear (see **Figure 5**), ileoanal pouch leakage, and rectal prolapse may all be diagnosed.

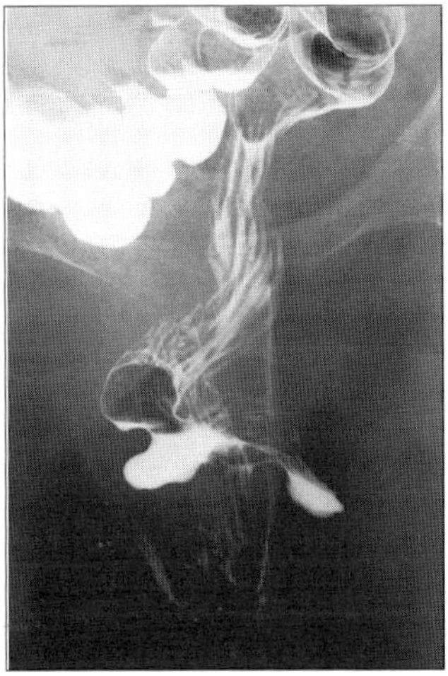

**Figure 3.** Lateral rectoceles demonstrated on dynamic proctography.

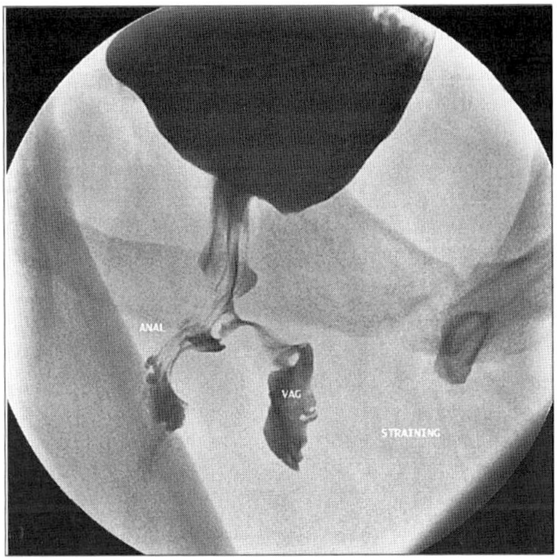


**Figure 4.** Oblique view of an anovaginal fistula seen on dynamic proctography.

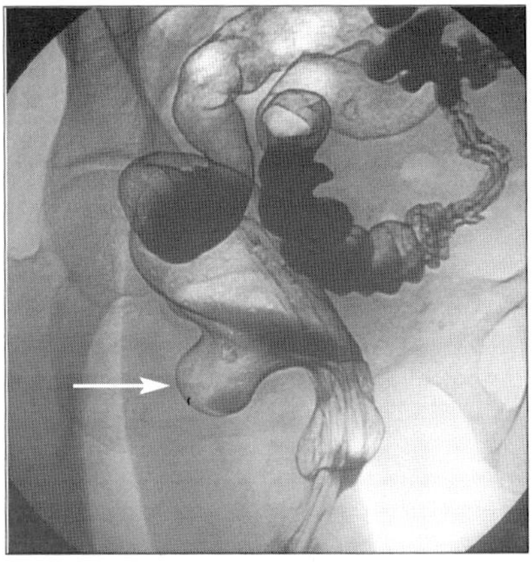

**Figure 5.** Pubococcygeal tear with herniation of rectal tissue (arrow) demonstrated on dynamic proctography. Hernia was only seen when the patient bore down with contrast in place during dynamic study.

## Complications

Patient discomfort and barium impaction.

## Additional comments

Dynamic proctography should be performed in a center where the staff have experience with the procedure. It is a time-consuming technique and the patient must be reassured and given clear instructions during the procedure to allow for optimal cooperation. Patient embarrassment during the procedure can produce radiographic changes mimicking nonrelaxing puborectalis syndrome.

# Chapter 2.7

# Electromyography

## Description of procedure

Anal electromyography (EMG) is the measurement of electrical activity in the anal muscle. The procedure involves placement of an electrode (using a needle, wire, or surface plug) onto the anal muscle. The electrical activity of the internal and external anal sphincter and the puborectalis muscles is then measured. Electrical action is measured at rest and during various maneuvers, including squeezing, pushing, and coughing (see **Figure 1**). The signal is transferred from the record electrode to an amplifier and oscilloscope. Data are converted via a computerized formula.

## Indications

Chronic constipation with suspected obstructive defecation disorders, chronic straining, suspected pelvic neuromuscular disorders, identification of anal sphincter injury, and fecal incontinence.

## Complementary procedures

Dynamic proctography, sigmoidoscopy, colonoscopy, sitz marker study, anorectal ultrasound, barium enema, and pudendal nerve terminal motor latency (PNTML).

## Contraindications

Bleeding disorders or anal carcinoma.

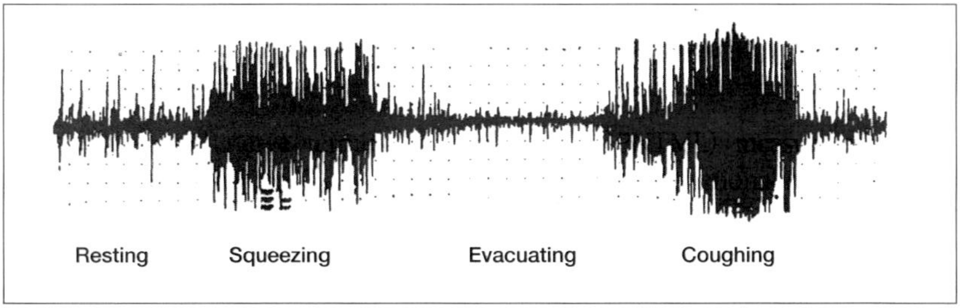


**Figure 1.** Normal EMG patterns with maneuvers.

## Relative contraindications

Inability to cooperate with testing, anal stenosis, anal abscess, or bleeding hemorrhoids.

## Preparation of patient

Some centers recommend a preparation of one or two sodium phosphate enemas just prior to the procedure; others do not recommend any enemas as preparation for the procedure.

## How the procedure is performed

Catheters may consist of a needle, a small single-fiber electrode, or a small anal plug made from a plastic or sponge material upon which surface electrodes have been mounted. After application of topical anesthesia, with the patient lying in a left lateral position, EMG catheters are inserted into the internal and external anal sphincters and puborectalis muscles. The catheters are connected to the amplifier and electrical transducer. Patients are instructed to perform various activities including squeezing, pushing (defecatory simulation), and coughing. Recordings are taken during these activities.

## Typical abnormal findings

EMG is highly effective for diagnosing nonrelaxing puborectalis syndrome and anismus. With these abnormalities, continued or increased muscle contraction occurs during a push maneuver. In anal sphincter injuries and neuromuscular damage, decreased or erratic motor function is documented.

## Complications

Patients often complain of discomfort; bleeding and/or infection are rare complications.

## Additional comments

Surface electrode techniques reduce patient discomfort and decrease the risk of infection; however, needle EMG is more accurate for documenting anal trauma and sphincter injuries. A 24-hour ambulatory EMG has been proposed as a sensitive means of correlating symptoms with disorders of the anal sphincter and puborectalis muscles. Surface electrode EMG has been used in biofeedback treatment of pelvic floor disorders.

# Chapter 2.8

# Flexible sigmoidoscopy

## Description of procedure

Flexible sigmoidoscopes are 8–12 mm in diameter and 60 cm in length. The sigmoidoscope is inserted into the anal canal and advanced proximally as far as patient tolerance permits. The flexible sigmoidoscope provides a well-lit, magnified view of the colonic mucosa. It has a suction channel to remove fecal material for analysis and a biopsy channel to obtain mucosal specimens for histologic analysis.

## Indications

Rectal bleeding, rectal mass, colitis, diarrhea, screening for colon cancer (in combination with stool Hemoccult® fecal blood testing), surveillance of patients with an ileoanal pouch, fecal incontinence (in combination with other studies), constipation (in combination with other studies), or screening of patients with a family history of familial polyposis syndromes.

## Complementary procedures

Barium enema, stool collection, Hemoccult® fecal blood test, anorectal ultrasound, anorectal manometry, and defecography.

## Contraindications

Imperforate anus.

## Relative contraindications

Severe anal or rectal pain (such as that caused by an anal fissure), anal or rectal stricture, or severe coagulopathy (in which biopsies should not be performed).

## Preparation of patient

The patient should only receive clear liquids after their dinner the night or 16 hours before the procedure and should be given two sodium phosphate enemas on the morning of the procedure. More aggressive preparations, such as 24 hours of clear liquids and oral laxatives, have been recommended by some to improve mucosal visualization. Some clinicians recommend flexible sigmoidoscopy without preparation in patients undergoing evaluation for colitis because a preparation may alter the appearance of the mucosa.

## How the procedure is performed

The patient is placed in a left lateral position and a gentle digital rectal examination is performed. It is important to perform a prostate examination on male patients at this time to screen for prostate cancer. The flexible sigmoidoscope is inserted and advanced to 60 cm, or as far as is tolerated by the patient. It is not uncommon for patient discomfort (due to sigmoid angulation and redundancy) to limit advancement of the flexible sigmoidoscope beyond 30 cm. If a large polyp is seen, the patient will undergo a colonoscopy for complete evaluation of the colon and removal of the polyp (see **Figure 1**). If smaller polyps are seen (see **Figures 2** and **3**), biopsies of these lesions are recommended. Colonoscopy is subsequently performed if adenomatous polyps are identified.

In patients with diarrhea caused by a suspected infection, fecal material may be suctioned and collected for culture, and ova, parasite, and *Clostridium difficile* toxin evaluation. Retroflexion of the sigmoidoscope in the distal rectum allows visualization of the proximal anal canal and the dentate line. This is particularly useful for looking at internal hemorrhoids and high anal canal lesions. The retroflexed view is also useful for finding polyps in the distal rectum (see **Figure 4**). If colitis is suspected based on visualization of the mucosa and/or clinical history, biopsies are obtained and sent for histologic evaluation.

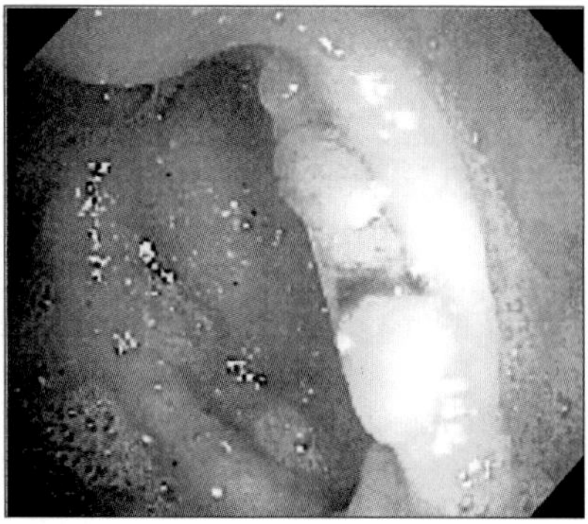

**Figure 1.** A large sessile sigmoid polyp. Removal will be technically challenging.

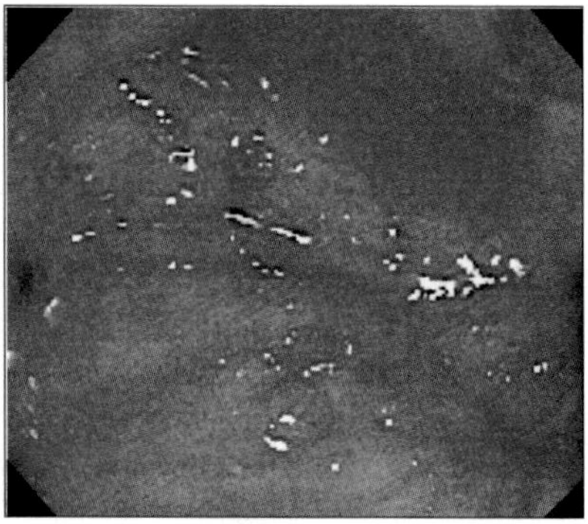

**Figure 2.** Small sessile rectal polyp, a common finding on flexible sigmoidoscopy.

## Typical abnormal findings

Screening of the distal 60 cm of the colon may reveal polyps or colon cancer, evaluation of the proximal 60 cm of the colon allows for identification of sources of rectal bleeding, including hemorrhoids and proctocolitis. Biopsies may be obtained for suspected colitis if the mucosal appearance is abnormal. Diverticulosis of the colon may also be identified (see **Figure 5**).

## Complications

Patient discomfort is common. Bleeding may occur subsequent to biopsies. Perforation is a very rare complication of flexible sigmoidoscopy.

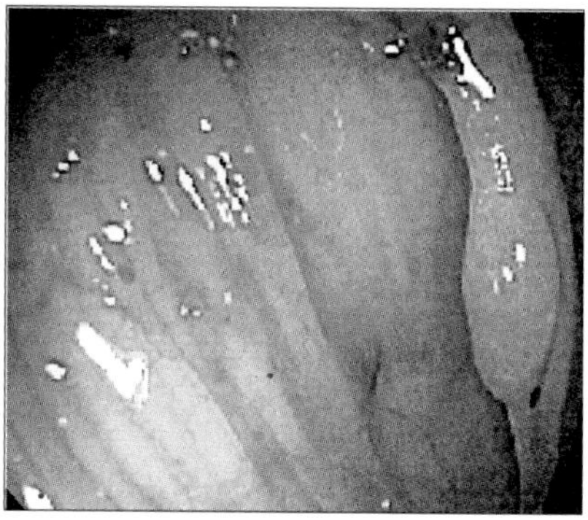

**Figure 3.** Sigmoid colon polyp demonstrated on flexible sigmoidoscopy.

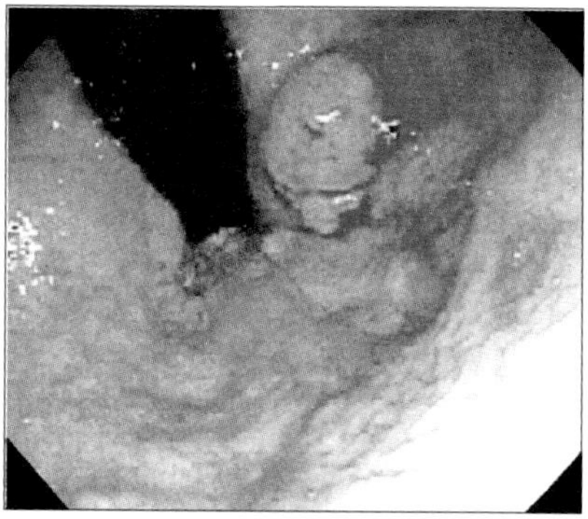

**Figure 4.** A sessile polyp near the dentate line seen on sigmoidoscopy.

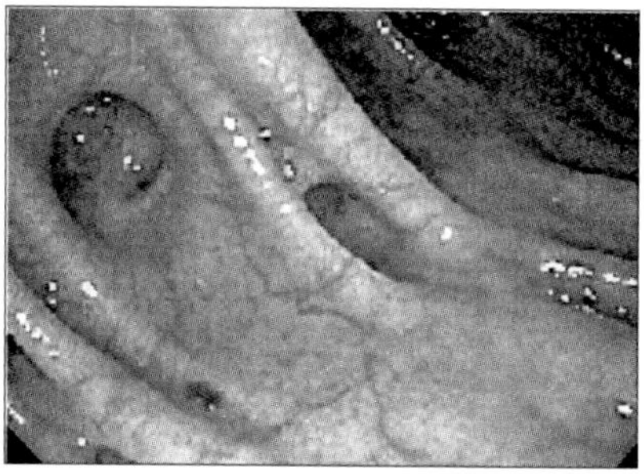

**Figure 5.** Sigmoid diverticulosis, a common endoscopic finding.

## Additional comments

In the United States, colonoscopy with visualization of the entire colon is replacing flexible sigmoidoscopy as the preferred method for screening for colon polyps and cancers.

# Chapter 2.9

# Pudendal nerve terminal motor latency

## Description of procedure

The pudendal nerve innervates the anal sphincters; therefore, pudendal nerve injury may result in sphincter dysfunction. Pudendal nerve terminal motor latency (PNTML) measures pudendal nerve function. With this procedure, a stimulating and recording electrode are utilized to measure the conduction of an impulse across the pudendal nerve.

## Indications

Fecal incontinence and chronic constipation.

## Complementary procedures

Anorectal ultrasound, anorectal manometry, defecography, and flexible sigmoidoscopy.

## Contraindications

Imperforate anus.

## Relative contraindications

A patient who is unable/unwilling to cooperate with the procedure.

## Preparation of patient

Some centers recommend a preparation of one or two Fleet's enemas prior to the procedure; others do not recommend any enemas as preparation for the procedure.

## How the procedure is performed

A physician places the electrode device over a gloved finger (a disposable model is available). This device has two stimulating electrodes at the tip of the gloved finger and two surface recording electrodes at the base of the finger. A grounding pad is applied to the patient's thigh. The finger is gently placed in the rectum with the tip of the finger pushing against the ischial spine. An electrical signal is given at the point of induction of contraction of the external anal sphincter, which may be felt by the examiner. The recording electrode then measures the latency separating the stimulating impulse and the contraction of the sphincter. This is termed the PNTML. Three readings are obtained at least three times on either side of the rectum. PNTML duration that is longer than $2.2 \pm 0.2$ ms is considered prolonged and is suggestive of pudendal nerve damage.

## Typical abnormal findings

Prolonged PNTML is seen in patients with unexplained fecal incontinence. Unfortunately, it also appears to occur as a natural consequence of aging. Prolonged PNTML has been associated with pudendal nerve damage due to pelvic floor laxity and rectal prolapse. Recent studies have failed to demonstrate a relationship between descent of the perineum (a potential cause of obstructive constipation) and prolongation of PNTML.

## Complications

None.

## Additional comments

This procedure is not recommended as a routine test in patients with chronic constipation or fecal incontinence due to a high rate of false positive results in these patients.

# Chapter 2.10

# Quantitative stool collection

## Description of procedure

In some patients with unexplained diarrhea, quantitative measurement of fecal volume, electrolytes, pH, and fat content over 24–72 hours will assist in determining the cause of diarrhea. Stools may be spot tested for occult blood, white blood cells, parasites, pathogenic bacteria, and *Clostridium difficile* toxin.

## Indications

Chronic diarrhea with or without weight loss and nutritional deficiencies.

## Complementary procedures

Colonoscopy with biopsy of the mucosa, upper endoscopy with small intestinal biopsy, complete blood count, serum chemistry, thyroid-stimulating hormone levels, stool culture, D-xylose serum test, 24-hour urine 5-hydroxyindole acetic acid (5-HIAA), small intestinal radiography, computed tomography scan of the abdomen and pelvis, and serum hormone levels (vasoactive intestinal peptide, gastrin, somatostatin, and calcitonin).

## Contraindications

None.

## Relative contraindications

Inability to collect stool specimens properly and to store over several days.

## Preparation of patient

For patients undergoing fecal fat testing, it is helpful to have a patient on a diet of 100 g fat per day. Patients should be given instructions regarding this diet. Patients should otherwise continue their usual activities.

## How the procedure is performed

All stools are collected over the designated time period using a special collection device that is placed over the toilet. Stools obtained during the collection period are stored in a sealed can containing a preservative. In between stool passages, the can with the collected stool is placed in a refrigerator. Patients keep a diary of all foods consumed during the collection period.

## Typical abnormal findings

The collected stool is measured for volume and weight. Diarrhea is considered to be present if the volume is >200 mL/day or the weight is >200 g/day (see **Table 1**). The following electrolytes are commonly measured: sodium (Na), potassium (K), chloride (Cl), magnesium (Mg), and bicarbonate ($HCO_3$). The fecal osmotic gap is calculated with the following formula:

**Fecal osmotic gap = 290 – 2(Na + K)**

| Stools | Secretory | Osmotic | Inflammatory |
|---|---|---|---|
| Weight (g/day) | >1000 | 500–1000 | <500 |
| Osmolality | n | + | n |
| Osmotic gap | n | + | n |
| Na, Cl | + | n | + |
| K, $HCO_3$ | low | n | n |
| pH | high | low | n |

**Table 1.** Stool features in chronic diarrhea. n: normal.

A fecal osmotic gap of <50 suggests secretory diarrhea, while a fecal osmotic gap of >100 is characteristic of osmotic diarrhea. A fecal pH of <6 is suggestive of a malabsorptive disorder. In normal individuals, the total amount of fat in the stool should be <6% of the amount consumed. Thus the presence of >6 g fat in the stool after consuming a 100 g fat diet suggests fat malabsorption. Very high fecal fat excretion (>20 g/day) is suggestive of pancreatic insufficiency. Elevated Mg in the stool can be found in laxative abusers. Additionally, the stool can be tested with a laxative screen using chromatography.

## Complications

None.

## Additional comments

Although this procedure may be beneficial in diagnosing difficult cases of unexplained diarrhea, quantitative stool collection is cumbersome and is strongly disliked by patients and laboratory personnel.

# Chapter 2.11

# Transanal ultrasound

## Description of procedure

This is a transanal procedure involving placement of an ultrasonographic probe into the anus and rectum. The device rotates 360° for full evaluation of the internal and external anal sphincters, as well as the rectum (compared to proctoscopy or sigmoidoscopy, which are used to view the mucosa only). Anorectal ultrasound has the advantage of evaluating all of the tissue layers of the examined organs.

## Indications

Evaluation of the anal sphincters in patients with fecal incontinence, staging of rectal cancers, evaluation of rectal lesions for evidence of invasion beyond the mucosa, and characterization of submucosal rectal lesions.

## Complementary procedures

Anorectal manometry, anorectal electromyography, defecography, flexible sigmoidoscopy, colonoscopy, and barium enema.

## Contraindications

Imperforate anus.

## Relative contraindications

Patient inability to cooperate with the procedure or severe anal stricture.

## Preparation of patient

The patient should receive two Fleet's enemas 1–3 hours before the procedure.

## How the procedure is performed

The patient is placed in a left lateral position. The ultrasonographic device is placed inside a hard plastic cover for evaluation of the anal canal, or inside a water-filled balloon for visualization of the rectum, and these are introduced into the anus. Ultrasound frequencies are transferred from the probe to a computer where they are reconstructed into a visual image. A resulting cross-sectional image of the anus and rectum is obtained. The internal anal sphincter appears as a dark ring surrounded by a whitish ring representing the external anal sphincter. The mucosa, submucosa, lamina propria, muscularis mucosa, and serosa of the rectum can all be visualized as separate layers.

## Typical abnormal findings

Transanal ultrasound can be used to evaluate the anatomy of the internal and external anal sphincter. Sphincter injuries (due to obstetric damage, trauma, and prior surgeries) can be visualized (see **Figure 1**). Thinning and degeneration of the anal sphincters may also be seen. The test may be used to evaluate patients who are being considered for sphincter repair for fecal incontinence. Transanal ultrasonography may be used to stage rectal carcinomas. Specifically, the test is accurate in determining whether the tumor is invading beyond the mucosa and the extent of this invasion. Enlargement of lymph nodes adjacent to the tumor may also be visualized. Therefore, this technique is useful in staging rectal tumors and for determining optimal medical and surgical management of the disease. Suspicious lymph nodes may also be sampled.

## Complications

Mild discomfort.

## Additional comments

This is an evolving technology. As with other forms of ultrasonography, the quality of information obtained from transanal ultrasonography is highly operator dependent.

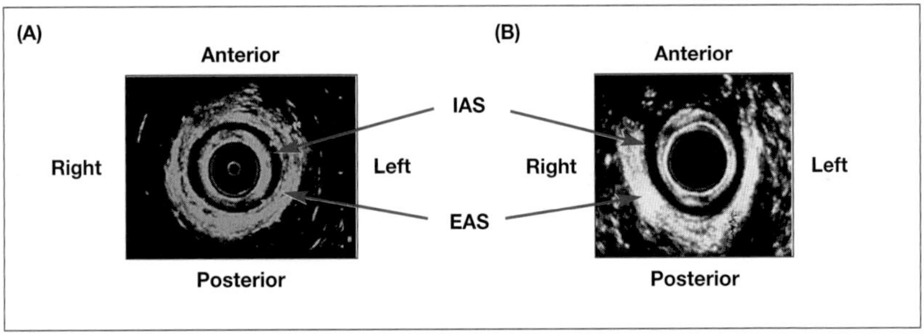


**Figure 1.** **(A)** Normal internal anal sphincter (IAS) and external anal sphincter (EAS); **(B)** anterior defect of IAS and EAS.

# Chapter 3

# Benign anorectal disorders

# Chapter 3.1

# Anal fissure

## Definition

A tear, crack, or ulceration of the anal canal.

## Epidemiology

An anal fissure can occur in any age group but is seen most commonly in young adults. They are found with equal frequency in males and females.

## Patients at risk

This condition may be brought on by the passage of a large, hard stool. It may occur more frequently in persons consuming low fiber, high fat diets. Anal fissures are also a feature of Crohn's disease, anorectal infections, leukemia, tuberculosis, and HIV infection.

## Pathophysiology

Anal fissures are most commonly seen in the posterior midline portion of the anal canal (see **Figure 1**). This area may have decreased blood flow due to the configuration of the vasculature of the anus. Spasm of the internal anal sphincter may cause further reduction in blood flow to the posterior anal canal. This region of the anal canal has a higher risk of tearing because the arrangement of the anal muscles leads to less well-developed support of the anoderm in this region. Patients with a chronic anal fissure also appear to have increased resting and

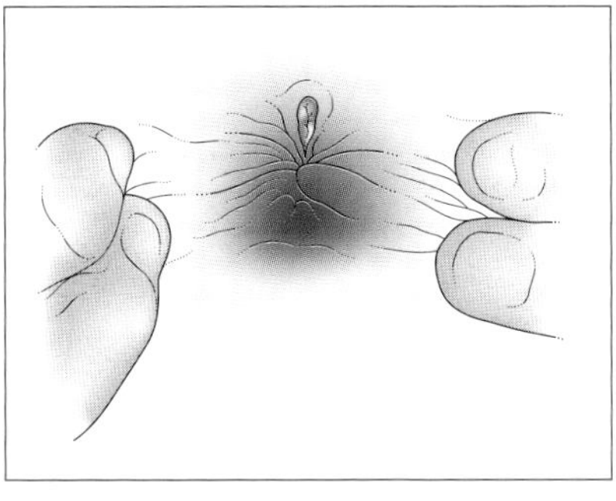

**Figure 1.** Large anal fissure as seen in typical posterior location (12 o'clock) on anal inspection.

contracting pressures in the anus. Many also experience an anal sphincter spasm on defecation.

## Symptoms

Pain and bleeding associated with defecation. The pain begins with defecation and persists after completion of the bowel movement. Bleeding is generally limited but may become severe and persistent.

## Diagnosis

External examination is usually sufficient to make a diagnosis. Most fissures are seen posteriorly, however, 25% of fissures in women and 8% of fissures in men are anterior. Gentle separation of the buttocks to expose the perianal area may facilitate examination. Some patients may experience extreme physical discomfort on examination and may require anesthesia prior to full evaluation. Occasionally, anoscopy or flexible sigmoidoscopy is utilized (although these procedures may result in significant discomfort to the patient and may also require anesthesia).

### Physical findings

1. Sentinel pile (a small skin tag located outside of the anal canal near the fissure).
2. The fissure itself.
3. Hypertrophied anal papilla (originating at the dentate line) (see **Figures 2** and **3**).

## Treatment

### Medical

First line: (45%–87% healing rate). Stool softeners, fiber supplements such as psyllium (6–12 g/day) or bran (10–15 g/day), local anesthetic agents (such as lidocaine, benzocaine, or pramoxine), or warm sitz baths. Relaxation and avoidance of straining when going to the bathroom may be beneficial.

Second line: (77%–92% healing rate). Application of 0.2% topical nitroglycerin – this must be specially compounded by the pharmacist from standard 2% nitroglycerin mixed with petroleum jelly or another vehicle (such as glycerin). Approximately 1 g (enough to cover the tip of a gloved finger) should be applied two to four times per day to the anus. Patients should stay recumbent on their left side for 10–15 minutes after application due to the risk of hypotension from systemic nitroglycerin absorption. Topical calcium channel blockers such as 0.2% nifedipine and 2% diltiazem have shown beneficial effects similar to topical nitroglycerin. These are currently not available in the United States.

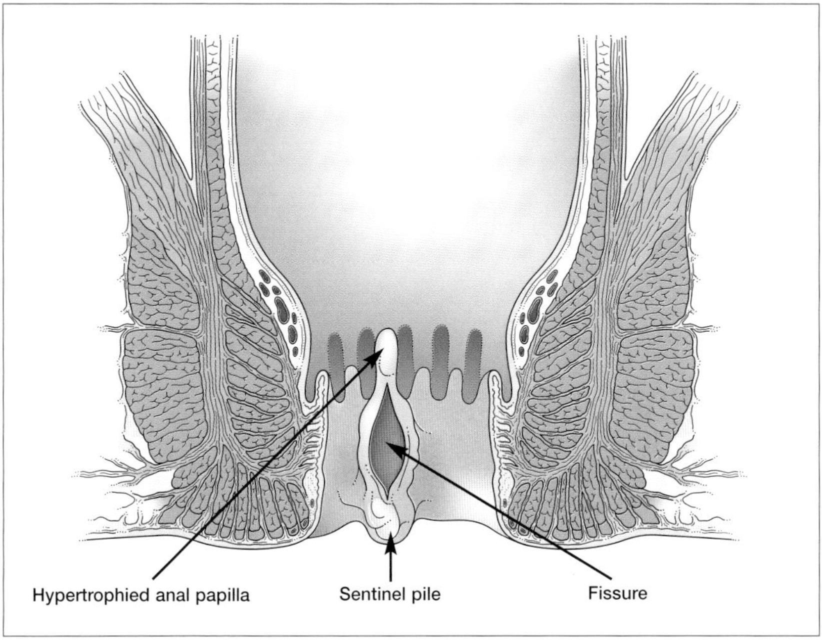


**Figure 2.** Classic anatomic findings in chronic anal fissure including sentinel pile, fissure, and hypertrophied anal papilla.

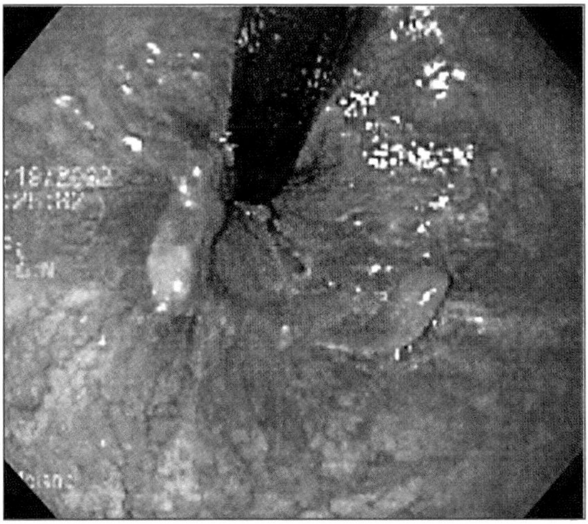

**Figure 3.** Endoscopic view of a chronic anal fissure and hypertrophied anal papilla.

Third line: (43%–100% healing rate). Botulinum toxin (Botox; 5–100 IU) may be injected into the internal anal sphincter using a small gauge needle and syringe.

A method for endoscopic delivery of Botox injections into the internal anal sphincter has been developed by our practice. An upper endoscope is used to view the dentate line. Betadyne is used to cleanse the area and Botox is then injected lateral to the dentate line.

### Surgical

Refractory patients require surgery. Surgical options include internal anal sphincterotomy with or without fissurectomy and manual dilatation of the anus, preferably in the operating room. These procedures carry the risk of the development of fecal incontinence: reported postoperative risk of incontinence is between 0%–38% with sphincterotomy and 8%–12% with anal dilatation.

## Clinical pearls

An anal fissure becomes chronic when an acute tear progresses to the development of frank ulceration. The use of topical nitroglycerin and Botox therapy has greatly enhanced the medical management of chronic anal fissures.

# Chapter 3.2

# Anal stenosis

## Definition

Narrowing of the anal canal.

## Epidemiology

Anal stenosis can be congenital, but this is rare. Most commonly, anal stenosis is an acquired disorder associated with a variety of conditions. The most common cause of anal stenosis is prior hemorrhoidectomy.

### Benign causes

Prior hemorrhoidectomy, fissurectomy, anal sphincter repair, rectovaginal fistula repair, electrocautery for anal condyloma, prior anorectal radiation therapy, rectal foreign body insertion, trauma, chronic diarrhea, excessive laxative or mineral oil use, and Crohn's disease.

### Malignant causes

Anal or rectal carcinoma.

## Pathophysiology

Excess anal skin utilization to close the wound after hemorrhoidectomy may cause stenosis. Carcinoma causes narrowing due to annular tumor growth. Scarring of the anus can occur secondary to Crohn's disease and as a complication of surgery. Excess anal skin utilization to close the wound after hemorrhoidectomy may cause stenosis. Laxative use and diarrhea may cause narrowing of the anal canal from anal sphincter hypertrophy. Normally, anal sphincter muscle function is preserved and muscular hypertrophy prevented by the presence of solid fecal boluses that intermittently cause dilatation and relaxation of the anal sphincter.

## Symptoms

Narrowing of the stool, passage of small stools, incomplete evacuation, painful defecation, and hematochezia (passage of red blood from the rectum) are symptoms of anal stenosis.

## Diagnosis

Diagnosis is via digital rectal examination. Difficulty of passage of the finger into the rectum occurs because of decreased anal diameter. Additional tests may include anoscopy, flexible sigmoidoscopy, colonoscopy, barium enema, or pelvic imaging, eg, a computed tomography (CT) scan. Biopsies are obtained to rule out malignancy. Anorectal ultrasound may improve visualization of the anal canal to rule out malignancy. Examination under anesthesia may be required.

## Treatment

### Medical

Bulking agents, stool softeners, and periodic dilatation using a digital method or flexible dilators of increasing diameter.

### Surgical

In cases of scarring, removal of the scar in combination with sphincterotomy. Anoplasty (the use of perianal skin to cover an area of the anal canal) is used for moderate–severe cases.

## Clinical pearls

In appropriately selected candidates, surgery appears to be the treatment of choice since stool bulking and anal dilatation are primarily temporizing and do not correct the narrowing of the anal canal.

# Chapter 3.3

# Anorectal abscess

## Definition

An infection that begins in the anal glands and extends into spaces around the anus and rectum.

## Epidemiology

Anorectal abscesses are most common in adults between the ages of 20 and 40 years. Twice as many males have this condition as females. Anorectal abscesses may occur in association with a variety of medical illnesses.

## Patients at risk

Anorectal abscesses are more common in patients with a variety of chronic medical conditions compared to the general population. Patients at risk include those with Crohn's disease, diabetes, heart disease, lymphoma, leukemia, anal and rectal cancer, radiation proctopathy, hidradenitis suppurativa, and infections of the perianal region. Anorectal abscesses can be caused by a variety of infections including, *Chlamydia* infection, actinomycosis, and tuberculosis.

## Pathophysiology

By definition, an anorectal abscess is a collection of pus in the perianal or perirectal region (see **Figure 1**).

The process is most likely initiated by obstruction of the anal glands followed by infections with the above-mentioned organisms or colonic bacteria. Infections may then expand into a variety of spaces within the anorectal region. The four most important locations where pus may accumulate are the perianal, ischiorectal, intersphincteric, and supralevator spaces (see **Figure 2**).

## Symptoms

The most common symptoms are pain and swelling in the anorectal region. Anal discharge and anorectal bleeding may be present.

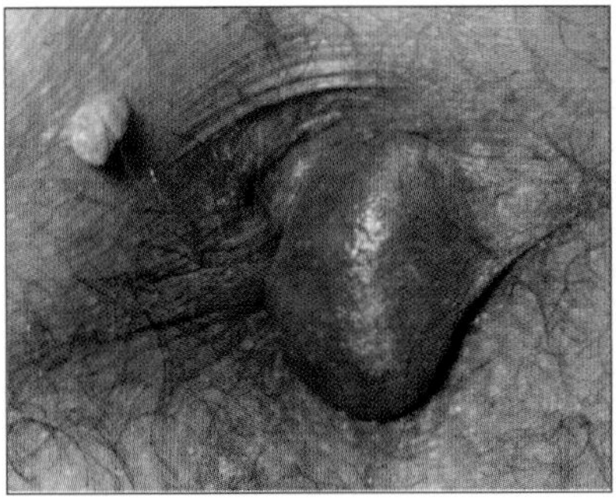

**Figure 1.** Perianal abscess with a small perianal wart opposite.

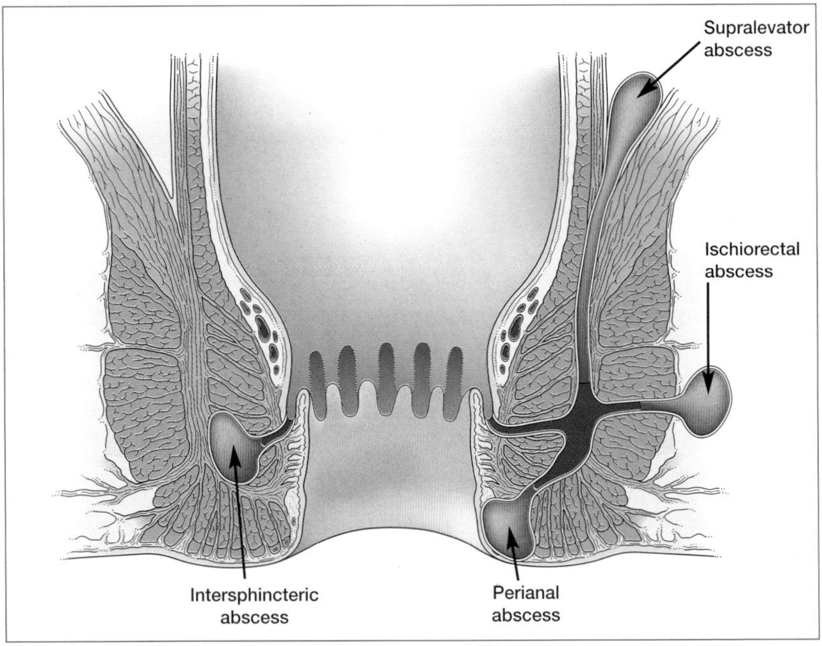


**Figure 2.** Classification of anorectal abscesses.

# Diagnosis

The diagnosis is made by taking appropriate history and physical examination. Examination reveals a swollen, tender, erythematous, warm enlargement in the perianal region. Some drainage may be present and a pin-like opening may be revealed. Anesthesia may be required to complete the examination, including a digital rectal evaluation.

## Treatment

All anorectal abscesses require drainage. This may be performed in the operating room or at the bedside depending on the location and severity of the abscess. Excision of a fistula associated with the abscess may be required at a later stage. Culturing of the material collected after drainage is suggested for individuals who are immunocompromised. Subsequent treatment with sitz baths, stool softeners, a high-fiber diet, laxatives, and local bandaging may be required. Treatment of the underlying disease is also beneficial.

## Clinical pearls

In routine cases of anorectal abscesses, preoperative and post-drainage antibiotics are only recommended in immunocompromised patients and individuals with valvular heart disease.

# Chapter 3.4

# Constipation

## Definition

This is a symptom most objectively defined as fewer than three spontaneous bowel movements per week. Other definitions include decreased stool bulk, change in stool caliber (diameter), and straining with stool passage.

## Epidemiology

Large national surveys in the United States including the National Health Interview Survey (NHIS) and the National Health and Nutrition Examination Survey (NHANES) suggest that between 2%–13% of the population of the United States report the symptom of constipation to their physician each year. According to the NHANES, 3.2% of males and 9.1% of females have fewer than three bowel movements per week. Studies in the United Kingdom suggest that the prevalence of constipation is between 8%–13%.

## Patients at risk

Constipation becomes more common with advancing age: prevalence in developed countries increases to 25% in the elderly. The rate of physician visits for the complaint of constipation increases from 1.3% for younger patients to 4.1% annually for persons over the age of 65 years. Symptoms of constipation are approximately three times more common in women than in men. Constipation appears to be more common in individuals of lower socioeconomic status and occurs less frequently in the white population.

## Pathophysiology

Causes of constipation may be divided into several categories, these are outlined below.

### Slow colonic transit

Decreased motility resulting from neuromuscular dysfunction. Causes include medications (anticholinergics, calcium channel blockers, opioids [see **Figure 1**]), Chagas' disease, Hirschsprung's disease, and endocrinopathies such as diabetes and hypothyroidism. Idiopathic colonic inertia is a syndrome seen predominantly in young women and may be due to a neuromyopathy.

### Obstructive defecation (pelvic floor disorders)

These may be due to anorectal muscle spasm (nonrelaxing puborectalis syndrome, anismus), prolapses (rectal prolapse, anorectal intussusception), rectoceles (see **Figures 2** and **3**), or pelvic laxity. These disorders are most commonly seen in women.

### Mechanical obstruction

Strictures (carcinoma, radiation-induced, Crohn's disease, diverticular, ischemic).

### Psychogenic

Patients may feel compelled to have daily bowel movements (due to an abnormal concern about having colonic disease).

## Symptoms

When daily bowel movements do not occur, patients may complain of decreased stool frequency, decreased stool bulk, narrow stools, and/or straining with stool passage.

## Diagnosis

### Laboratory

Complete blood count, thyroid stimulating hormone, and serum electrolytes.

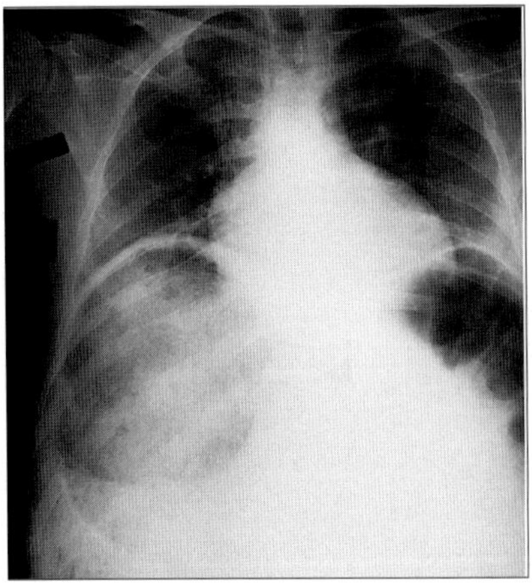

**Figure 1.** Abdominal plain radiograph demonstrates dilated left and right colon in a patient on chronic opioid therapy.

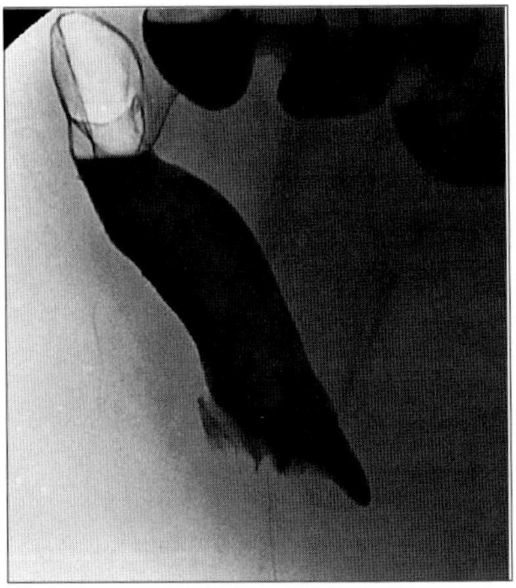

**Figure 2.** Rectocele demonstrated on dynamic proctography.

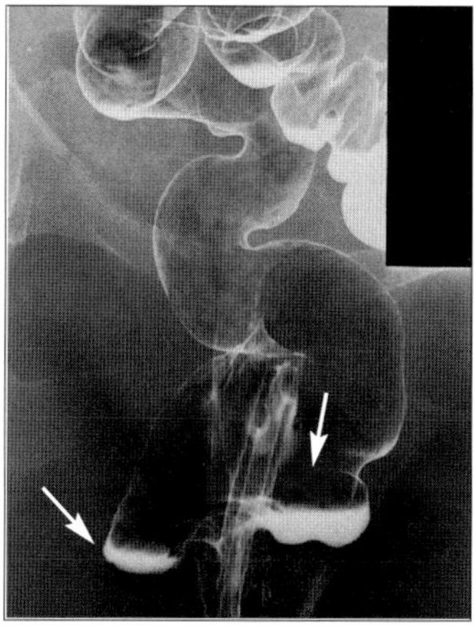

**Figure 3.** Lateral rectoceles (arrows) demonstrated on dynamic proctography. Patient complained of difficulty with evacuation.

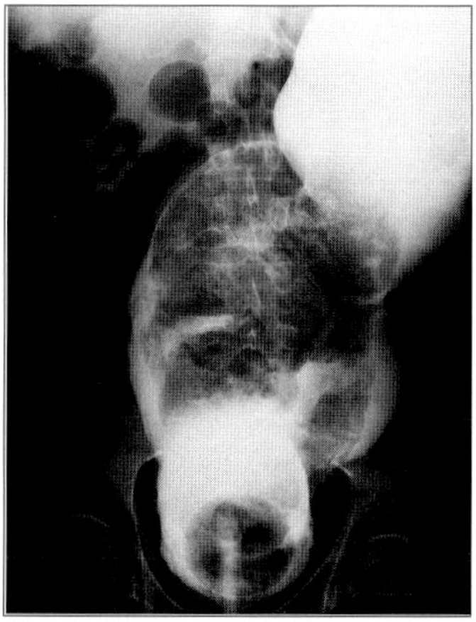

**Figure 4.** Megarectum demonstrated on barium enema in a patient with chronic constipation.

### Anatomic

Colonoscopy, barium enema (see **Figure 4**), flexible sigmoidoscopy, or anoscopy.

### Physiologic (obstructive defecation)

Dynamic proctography, anorectal manometry, nerve conduction velocity, electromyography, and sitz marker study (see **Figures 5–7**).

### Other

Full thickness rectal biopsy (in patients with suspected Hirschsprung's disease).

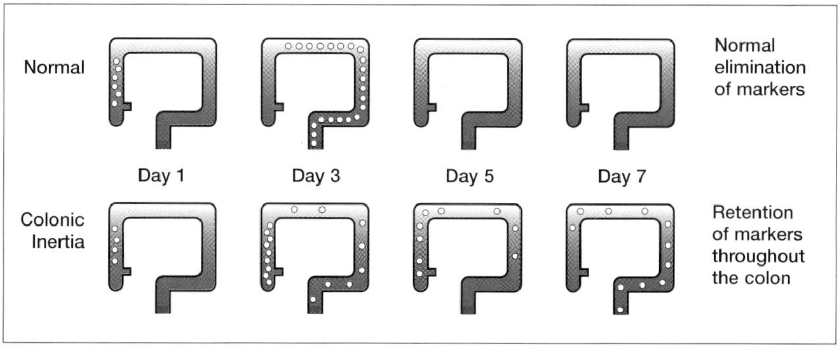


**Figure 5.** Movement of sitz markers in the colon in normal subjects and patients with colonic inertia. Patients with colonic inertia have accumulation of markers throughout the colon on day 5 after ingestion.

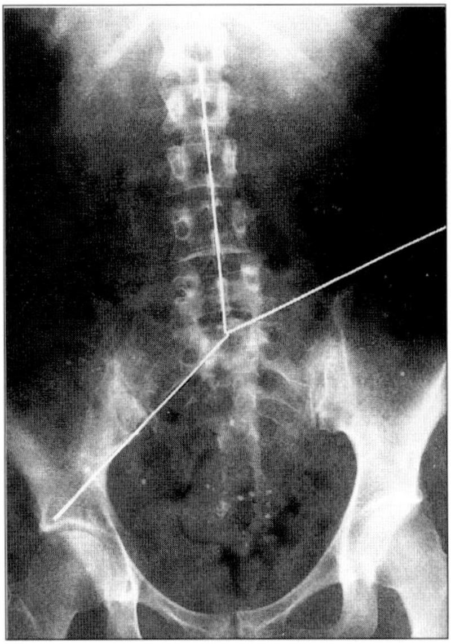

**Figure 6.** Sitz marker study on day 5 in a constipated patient demonstrates markers throughout the colon. Lines separate the right, middle, and left colon. Marker distribution patterns vary depending on the cause of constipation.

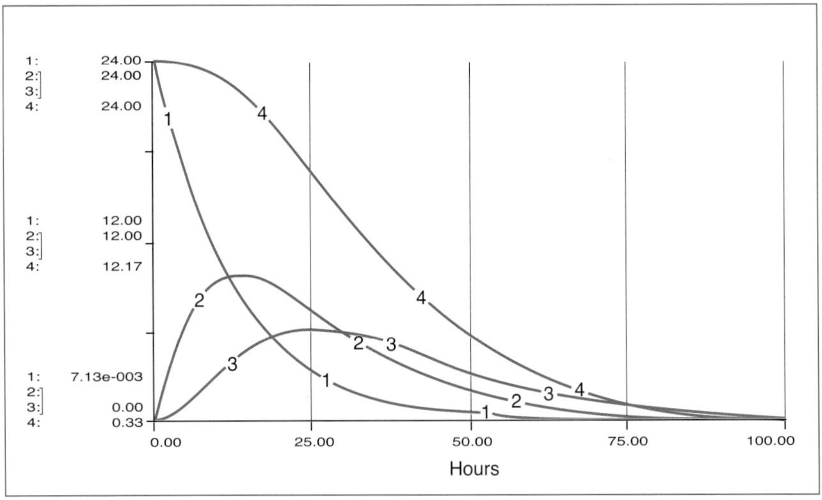


**Figure 7.** Simulation of segmental colonic transit of sitz markers based on data from 20 normal volunteers (1: right colon; 2: left colon; 3: rectosigmoid colon; 4: colon).

## Treatment

Fiber therapy, laxatives, stool softeners, lactulose and sorbitol, polyethylene glycol plus electrolytes, biofeedback therapy, botulinum toxin (Botox) injections, surgical repair of rectocele, subtotal colectomy and ileorectal anastomosis for colonic inertia, and lateral internal anal sphincterotomy.

## Clinical pearls

Taking a careful history will assist in differentiating the various causes of constipation. In general, an anatomic evaluation of the large intestine with a barium enema or colonoscopy should be included in the evaluation to screen for colon polyps, colonic strictures, and malignancies.

# Chapter 3.5

# Fecal incontinence

## Definition

Inadvertent passage of rectal contents, including soiling of underclothing or involuntary passage of gas, mucus, or liquid/solid stool.

## Epidemiology

Incontinence may be defined as gas incontinence, liquid incontinence, or formed stool incontinence. Episodic incidents occur in 2%–7% of surveyed individuals in the United States and Europe. Frank incontinence of solid stool is more rare and is seen in 0.7% of surveyed individuals in the United States and Europe. Fecal incontinence is most common in older women, and is the second most common cause of nursing home placement in the elderly. About 25% of patients with diarrhea-predominant irritable bowel syndrome have episodes of fecal incontinence. Patients often avoid reporting the symptom of fecal incontinence.

## Patients at risk

The elderly, patients with neurologic disease or injury, prior anorectal surgery, prior anorectal obstetric trauma, receptive traumatic anal intercourse, other anorectal trauma, colitis, chronic diarrhea, fecal impaction, or congenital anomalies.

## Pathophysiology

Incontinence occurs when normal anorectal function is disrupted. Damage to the anal sphincter, diseases of sensory and motor neurons of the pelvis, altered sensorium, and spinal cord injury may all result in leakage of stool due to inadequate sensation of the presence of stool in the rectum. Fecal soiling may occur in the elderly from constipation and overflow incontinence (involuntary loss of urine due to overdistention of the bladder).

## Symptoms

Classification by the type of incontinence and severity is important for determining the treatment regimen. Classification should be made on the basis of the factors shown in **Table 1**.

| | |
|---|---|
| Contents | Gas, liquid, or solid stool |
| Frequency | Rare, occasional, usual, or constant |
| Wearing of a pad | Rare, occasional, usual, or constant |
| Effects on lifestyle | Mild, moderate, or severe |

**Table 1.** Factors determining severity of incontinence type.

## Diagnosis

Digital rectal examination to identify resting tone and sphincter deformities; anorectal manometry to measure resting and squeeze pressures; anorectal ultrasound to visualize the sphincter for injury or other deformities; electromyography (EMG) and pudendal nerve terminal motor latency (PNTML) for detecting neuromuscular damage.

## Treatment

### Medical

- Antidiarrheal agents including loperamide, diphenoxylate, codeine, and other opiates
- Anticholinergic agents including hyoscyamine, dicyclomine, atropine, and clindium
- Fiber supplements, particularly calcium polycarbophyl
- Other constipating agents including cholestyramine
- Performance of Kegel exercises
- Biofeedback therapy

### Procedural

A new system called Secca® (Curon Medical) (see **Figure 1**) utilizes the delivery of radiofrequency waves into the anal sphincter. The technique results in remodeling of sphincter muscles and appears to improve symptoms.

### Surgical

Anorectal muscle repair; gracilis muscle transposition; gracilis muscle transposition with neuromuscular stimulation; artificial sphincter production; colostomy.

## Clinical pearls

Daily laxatives combined with enema therapy once per week have been shown to effectively reduce incontinence episodes in elderly patients with overflow incontinence.

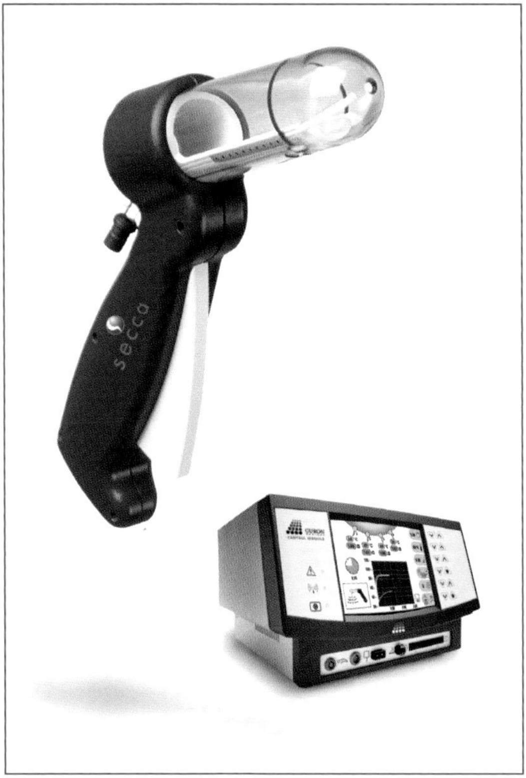


**Figure 1.** The Secca System for treatment of fecal incontinence.

# Chapter 3.6

# Hemorrhoids

## Definition

Dilation of anal venous structures.

## Epidemiology

Hemorrhoids occur in up to 50% of the adult population.

## Anatomy

### Internal

Internal hemorrhoids are dilatations of the venous structures in the internal hemorrhoidal plexus (see **Figure 1**). The veins are lined with rectal mucosa (transitional and columnar epithelium), which contains limited pain fibers. Internal hemorrhoids originate from above the dentate line (see **Chapter 1.1: Anal and rectal anatomy**).

### External

External hemorrhoids arise from the inferior venous plexus. It is lined up with the perianal squamous endothelium and contains a large number of pain fibers. External hemorrhoids originate from below the dentate line (see **Figure 2**).

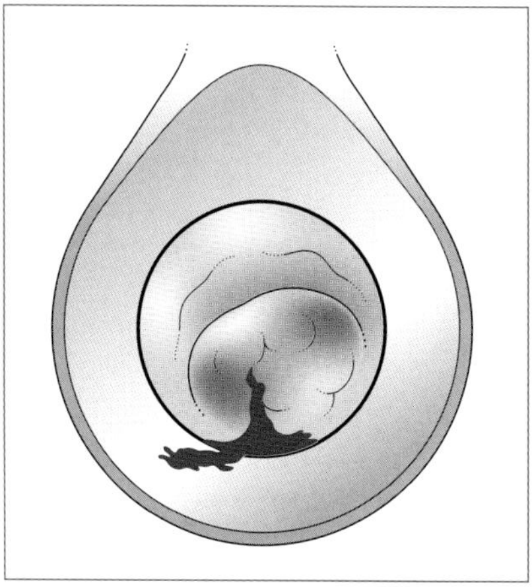

**Figure 1.** Internal hemorrhoid as seen on anoscopy.

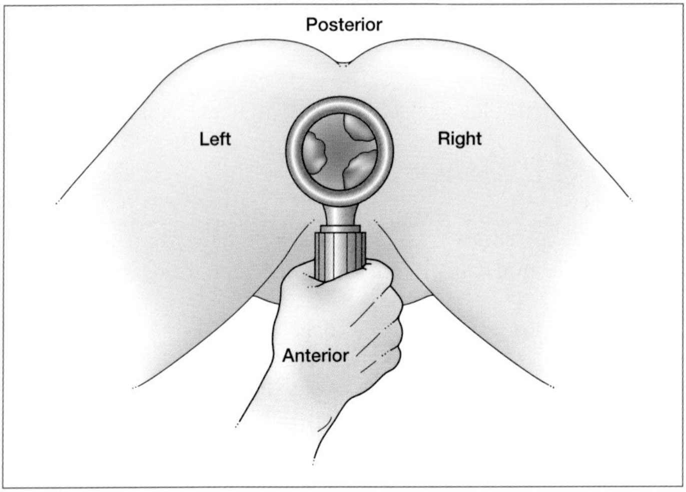


**Figure 2.** The main locations of internal hemorrhoids: right anterior, right posterior, and left lateral.

## Patients at risk

The elderly and those with straining secondary to chronic constipation, pregnancy, pelvic malignancy, chronic obstructive pulmonary disease with chronic cough, chronic diarrhea, and a variety of diseases or syndromes that increase the venous pressure within the pelvis.

## Pathophysiology

Hemorrhoids are made up of blood vessels, connective tissue, and lining tissue (rectal or anal mucosa). Aging and straining reduce the ability of the connective tissue to provide adequate support for hemorrhoids resulting in their dilatation and decreased venous return. Inflammation of overlying mucosa may contribute to symptomatology.

## Complications

### Internal hemorrhoids

Bleeding.

First-degree prolapse: internal hemorrhoids move into the anal canal.

Second-degree prolapse: prolapse of hemorrhoids outside the anal canal with straining, which resolves spontaneously.

Third-degree prolapse: hemorrhoids protrude outside of the anal canal and require replacement by digital maneuvers.

Fourth-degree prolapse: hemorrhoids protrude outside the anal canal and cannot be manually reduced.

### External hemorrhoids

Thrombosis: by definition, this occurs when a clot is present in an external hemorrhoid (see **Figure 3**). Secondary inflammation, bleeding, and ulceration may follow.

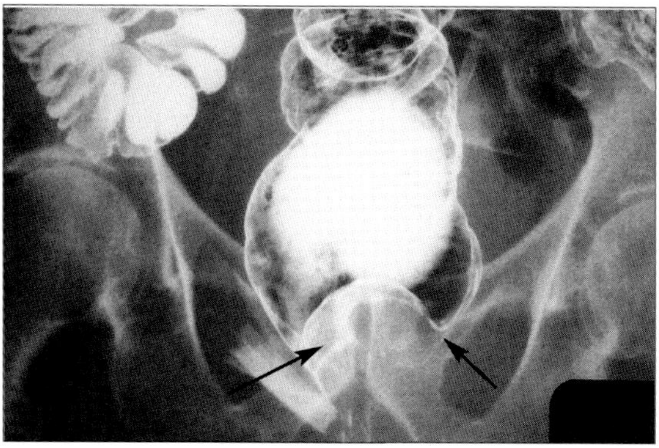

**Figure 3.** Thrombosed hemorrhoid. Rare barium study demonstrates filling defect (arrows).

## Symptoms

### Internal hemorrhoids

Sensation of prolapse, mild discomfort, soiling, passage of small quantities of bright red blood. Severe pain associated with prolapse may suggest strangulation of prolapsed internal hemorrhoids. This is a serious, potentially life-threatening condition.

### External hemorrhoids

Pain (primarily with thrombosis). Presence of external skin tag and pruritus ani.

## Diagnosis

Perianal examination. Prolapse may be demonstrated by having the patient perform a straining maneuver. Gentle palpation is used to diagnose thrombosis of external hemorrhoids. Anoscopy or sigmoidoscopy is required to diagnose internal hemorrhoids that are not prolapsed.

# Treatment

## General

Internal hemorrhoids: a high-fiber diet, increased fluids, and avoidance of straining. Add fiber supplements such as psyllium (Metamucil, Konsyl), methylcellulose (Citrucel), or calcium polycarbophyl (FiberCon). Sitz baths relieve discomfort.

External hemorrhoids: when thrombosis is present, sitz baths are recommended three to four times per day and after each bowel movement. A high-fiber diet, stool softeners, fiber supplementation as above, and laxatives may be beneficial. Patients should avoid straining. Topical local anesthetic creams (such as lidocaine, benzocaine, or pramoxine) should be applied two to four times per day.

## Nonsurgical, procedural

These treatments are utilized for internal hemorrhoids only. They are most effective for first- and second-degree prolapsed hemorrhoids.

Rubber band ligation: this is an outpatient procedure performed after placement of an anoscope. A specialized device grabs the hemorrhoid and places a rubber band tightly around it (see **Figure 4**). Complications associated with this technique include pain (sometimes resulting in the need to remove the rubber band), bleeding from early dislodgment of the rubber bands, infection, and perirectal abscess. Severe necrotizing infection from gas-forming organisms is a very rare reported complication.

Injection: this is a form of sclerotherapy using a sclerosing agent. The chemical is injected near the hemorrhoids causing an inflammatory reaction and a clot within the hemorrhoid. Complications associated with this technique include infection, ulceration, and pain.

Photocoagulation: this method uses infrared light to produce venous thrombosis and scarring. This technique is easily performed as an outpatient procedure without sedation and is well tolerated. Complications associated with this technique include pain and ulceration.

Other methods: cryosurgery, electrocoagulation, and saline injections.

## Surgical

Internal hemorrhoids: most proctologists agree that third- and fourth-degree hemorrhoids require hemorrhoidectomy. Stapled hemorrhoidectomy has been recently introduced and involves the use of circular staples applied above

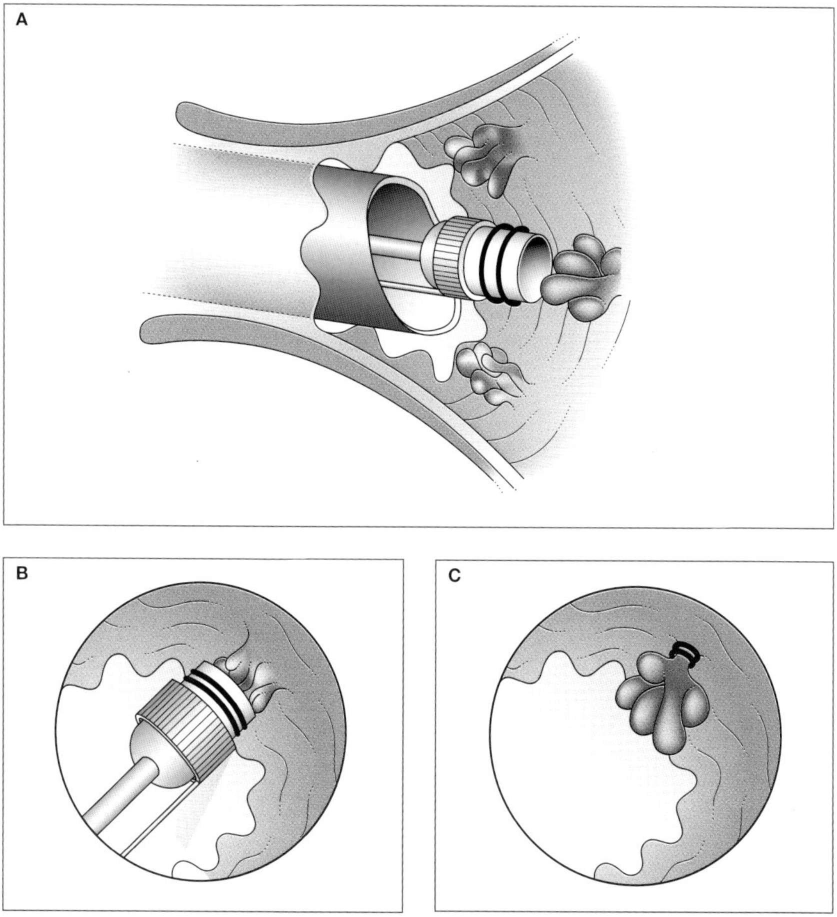


**Figure 4.** Technique for rubber band ligation of internal hemorrhoids. **(A)** The aspirator-ligator is inserted through an anoscope. **(B)** Suction is applied, pulling the mucosa and venous plexus into the suction cup. **(C)** The ligator is fired and two rubber bands are applied. Only one or two areas are banded in a single session.

(proximal to) the dentate line. Early studies have shown that this technique is associated with less postoperative pain than conventional hemorrhoidectomy.

External hemorrhoids: surgery is utilized in patients who have pain that is severe and/or lasts >48 hours. Treatment involves either removal of the thrombosis or excision of the hemorrhoid. Thrombectomy alone cannot be performed after approximately 48 hours.

## Clinical pearls

It is important to differentiate hemorrhoids from anorectal varices, which occur in patients with pre-existing portal hypertension. Like external hemorrhoids, anorectal varices begin below the dentate line then expand into the rectum. Bleeding anorectal varices are most often treated with nonsurgical procedures such as rubber band ligation, as described for internal hemorrhoids.

# Chapter 3.7

# Hidradenitis suppurativa

## Definition

An acute or chronic inflammatory and infectious disorder of the apocrine (sweat) glands. It often occurs in the perianal, inguinal, or genital areas.

## Epidemiology

This condition most commonly occurs in younger individuals, between the ages of 16–45 years. It is more common in women. However, perineal involvement requiring surgery appears to be more common in men.

## Patients at risk

This condition is closely associated with Crohn's disease. It is more common in blacks than whites. Predisposing conditions include diabetes mellitus, seborrhea, and obesity.

## Pathophysiology

The process is initiated when an apocrine duct becomes obstructed by keratinous secretions. This results in expansion of the sweat gland and secondary infection from skin flora and colonic bacteria. Rupture of the gland leads to involvement of adjacent areas and spreading of the infection (see **Figure 1**). The most common site of involvement is the axilla. The next most commonly involved sites are the perianal and genital regions. Poor skin hygiene and a prior history of acne may predispose to the development of the condition.

## Symptoms

Patients develop pruritus, pain, and leakage from the affected area.

## Diagnosis

Physical examination reveals multiple lesions at affected sites. Lesions are erythematous and tender to palpation. A purulent discharge may be present. Extensive sinus formation with palpable abscesses and a honeycomb-like distribution of the lesions may be seen in the region of the anus, genitalia, gluteus, and thighs.

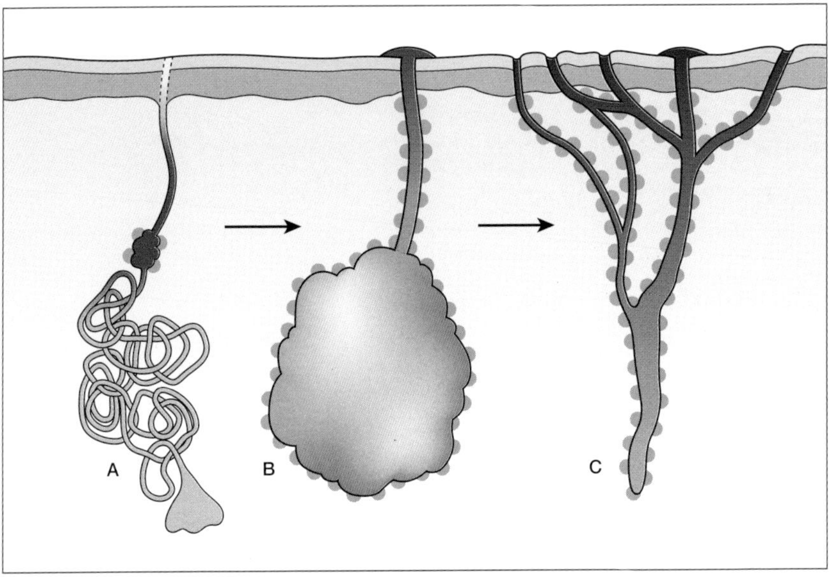


**Figure 1.** Hidradenitis suppurativa. **(A)** The first event is blockage of an apocrine duct by a keratinous plug. **(B)** Bacteria trapped beneath the plug multiply to form an abscess, with rupture into adjacent tissue. **(C)** Subsequently, recurrent abscesses, draining sinuses, and indurated scarred skin and subcutaneous tissues occur.

## Treatment

Cleansing of affected areas may be beneficial. Discontinuation of oral contraceptive therapy has been effective in some patients.

Antibiotic therapy with coverage for skin and colon flora may be effective in early disease. Suitable antibiotics include tetracycline, erythromycin, Augmentin (amoxicillin/clavulanate potassium), and penicillin. Oral isotretinoin has been effective in a small number of patients. Topical clindamycin has also been helpful, as have topical and intralesional injections with steroids. Surgical management for nonresponsive patients involves excision of the sinuses, sometimes with application of a graft to the surgical wound.

## Clinical pearls

Hidradenitis suppurativa may be confused with infections of the perianal region, sebaceous cysts, and perianal Crohn's disease.

# Chapter 3.8

# Nonrelaxing puborectalis syndrome

*(Also known as: anismus, paradoxical puborectalis contraction)*

## Definition

Inability to defecate due to spasm of the puborectalis muscle and other components of the anal sphincter.

## Epidemiology

There is no information on the epidemiology of this condition; however, clinical experience suggests that this is a relatively uncommon disorder. It appears to occur more frequently in individuals over the age of 50 years.

## Patients at risk

This condition may be associated with anxiety and obsession regarding bowel habits. Patients with a history of sexual abuse appear to be at higher risk for developing the condition, however, the reason for this is unknown.

## Pathophysiology

The puborectalis muscle attaches to the pubic bone and envelops the distal rectum in a sling-like fashion, forming the anorectal angle. It is a skeletal muscle, which is normally in a contracted state at rest. The anorectal angle assists with maintaining continence. The puborectalis muscle relaxes at the time of defecation, thus increasing the anorectal angle, allowing stool to move distally for evacuation. People with this condition are unable to relax the puborectalis muscle and external anal sphincter, thus developing a form of pelvic floor obstruction and constipation.

## Symptoms

Difficulty with evacuation, straining, and incomplete evacuation are the most common symptoms. The passage of multiple small stools with marked straining may also suggest this diagnosis.

## Diagnosis

Physical examination with digital rectal examination may reveal the diagnosis. Patients are asked to push to assist evacuation of the finger within the rectum. Lack of relaxation of the sphincter with this maneuver may suggest the presence of nonrelaxing puborectalis syndrome. However, a number of authors have cautioned that this physical finding is only suggestive of the diagnosis. Anorectal manometry, dynamic proctography, and anorectal electromyography (EMG) are the most useful diagnostic tests for this condition. Some authors have suggested that dynamic proctography and anorectal manometry should both be performed if the nonrelaxing puborectalis syndrome is suspected since each test performed individually lacks sensitivity and specificity.

## Treatment

Patient education may be of some benefit. Fiber supplementation is beneficial, and injection of 6–15 IU of botulinum toxin (Botox) into the puborectalis muscle or external anal sphincter region has recently been shown to be successful in a small number of patients. Biofeedback therapy has proven to be beneficial in up to 90% of patients. Surgical management may be an option for some patients; however, only a limited number of surgical studies has been performed. For example, a small group of patients appears to have benefited from lateral division of the puborectalis muscle. A small number of patients also appears to have benefited from dilatation of the anal sphincter with dilators of increasing diameter.

## Clinical pearls

Sphincter nonrelaxation on anorectal manometry and defecography may occur in patients who are excessively nervous when undergoing these procedures. Our group has demonstrated a beneficial effect of Botox injection into the internal anal sphincter via an endoscopic route for patients with spasmic anorectal disorders. Nonrelaxing puborectalis syndrome is not associated with anorectal pain. It is important to consider the diagnosis of levator ani syndrome in patients complaining of pain and difficulty with evacuation. Patients with levator ani syndrome will have marked tenderness of the anal sphincter on digital rectal examination.

# Chapter 3.9

# Perianal Crohn's disease

## Definition

The development of a variety of pathologic conditions of the perianal region such as fistulas, abscesses, and strictures caused by inflammation from Crohn's disease (see **Figure 1**).

## Epidemiology

Perianal symptoms occur in more than 40% of patients with Crohn's disease. Perianal pathology includes the development of fistulas, anal fissures, and abscesses. Perianal fistulas are seen in 28% of patients with Crohn's disease. Enlarged, thickened anal skin tags are frequently present and form *de novo* as a direct effect of local inflammation (see **Figure 2**).

## Patients at risk

Perianal involvement is more common in patients with rectal Crohn's disease (92%) and colonic Crohn's disease (52%) than in those with small intestinal Crohn's disease (14%). Patients with Crohn's proctitis are at particular risk for perianal fistulas. A symptomatic perianal fistula is the initial clinical presentation in about 5% of patients with Crohn's disease.

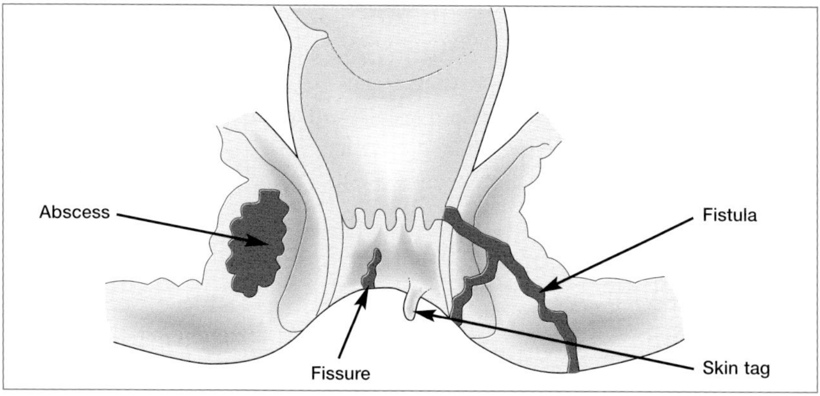


**Figure 1.** Anorectal disorders seen in patients with Crohn's disease.

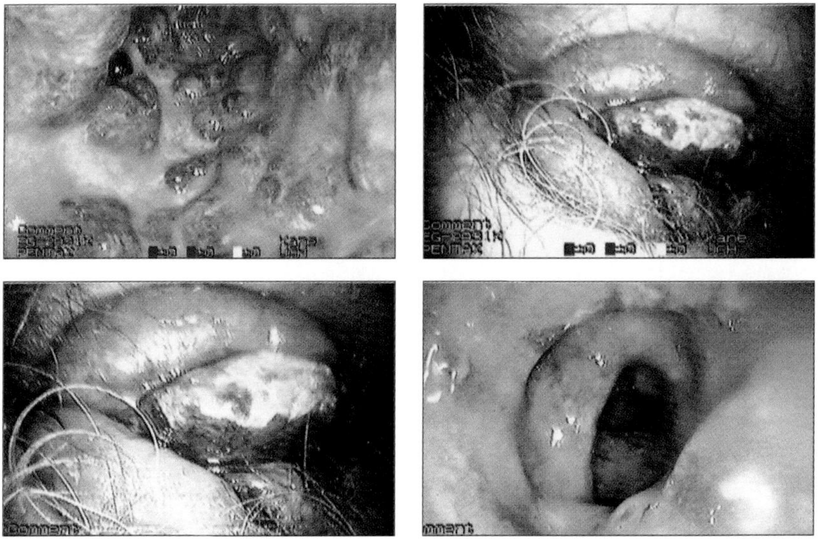

Figure 2. Perianal Crohn's disease with large skin tags, perianal inflammation, proctitis, and thrombosed hemorrhoids (photo courtesy of Dr Sunanda V Kane).

## Pathophysiology

Transmural, chronic inflammation of the gut wall extends to local tissues. Secretion of proteases and other destructive enzymes results in the development of sinus cavities. Anal gland inflammation extends into adjacent tissues, which results in anal fistulization and abscess formation. Secondary infection within these spaces occurs due to exposure to colonic bacteria. Complex fistulas are a distinguishing feature of perianal Crohn's disease.

## Symptoms

About 25% of patients with perianal Crohn's disease are asymtomatic or require no treatment. Pruritus ani and mild discomfort after the passage of stool occur in some patients. When abscesses are present, pain, fever, and systemic symptoms may occur. A system for classification of severity has been developed based on the amount of pain, limitation of activity, restriction of sexual activity, type of perianal involvement, and degree of induration.

## Diagnosis

Physical examination reveals enlarged anal skin tags (termed "elephant ears"), perianal openings due to fistulization, induration of the surrounding skin, anal abscesses, and anal strictures. Patients may have complex perianal involvement with ulceration and multiple fistula tracks. Extension to the labia, scrotum, thigh, groin, and buttocks may be present (see **Figures 3–5**). Testing may include the use of computed tomography (CT), magnetic resonance imaging (MRI), anorectal ultrasound, or fistulography as clinically indicated.

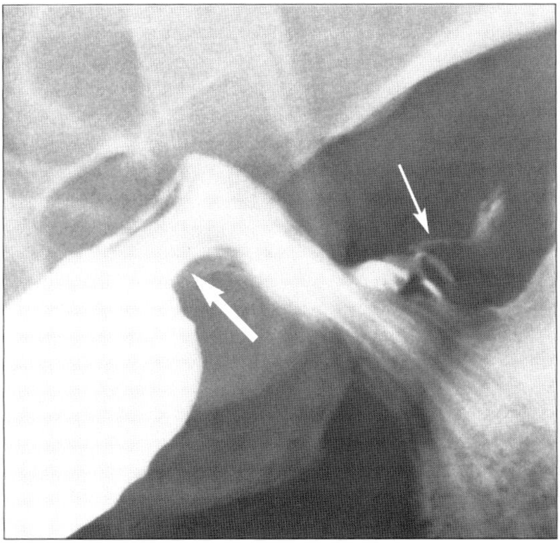

**Figure 3.** Lateral view of an anovaginal fistula (small arrow) in a patient with Crohn's disease. Spasm of the puborectalis muscle is noted (large arrow).

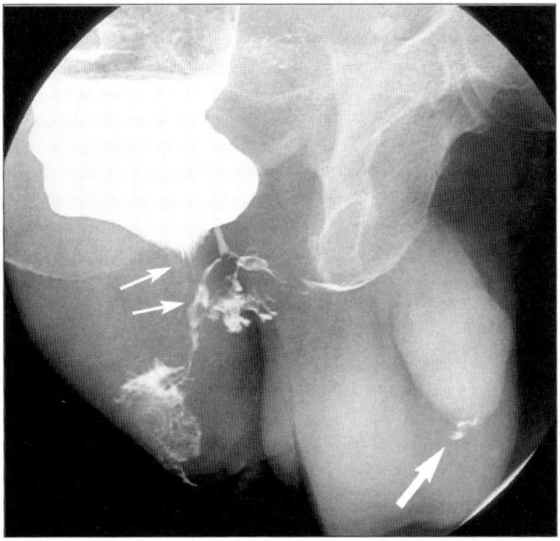

**Figure 4.** Anal urethral fistula (arrows) in a male patient with perianal Crohn's disease. A small quantity of contrast is seen exiting the penis from the urethra meatus (large arrow).

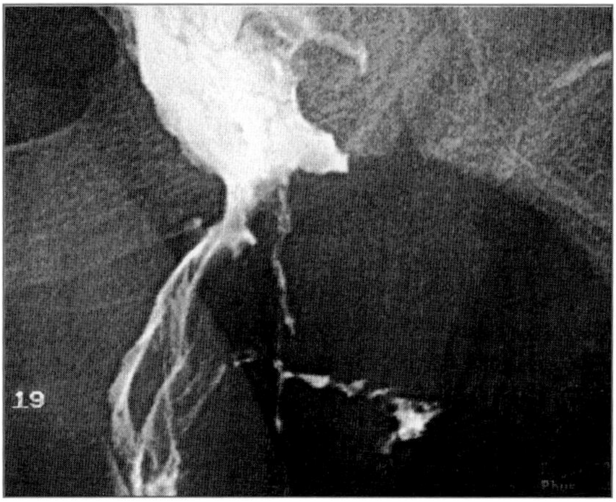


**Figure 5.** Fistulization from the perianal region to the thigh and gluteal areas in a patient with longstanding Crohn's disease.

# Treatment

## Medical

Medical therapy for Crohn's disease may also be suitable for the perianal complications of the disease. Immunosuppressants, including 6-mercaptopurine and azathioprine, may induce healing of perianal disease. Antibiotic therapy, particularly metronidazole has been found to be beneficial. Recently, infliximab (Remicade) has been shown to be highly effective in healing perianal fistulas.

## Surgical

Approximately 4% of patients with Crohn's disease require surgery for perianal disease. Surgical management includes incision and drainage of perianal and perirectal abscesses, placement of draining devices such as setons, and modified fistulotomy with or without an advancement flap. Some patients with severe perianal Crohn's disease will require a diverting ileostomy or a proctectomy and permanent ileostomy placement.

# Clinical pearls

Although rare, perianal carcinoma is a known complication of perianal Crohn's disease. Marked changes in symptomatology should prompt a careful investigation, including possible examination under anesthesia. Fistulous surgery must be carefully performed in the setting of active Crohn's disease as prolonged difficulties with wound healing may occur as a complication of surgery.

Decisions regarding surgical management depend on the presence or absence of active Crohn's disease in other portions of the bowel, whether Crohn's disease is involving the rectum, and whether complex fistulas are present.

# Chapter 3.10

# Perianal fistula

## Definition

A pathologic connection between the anal canal and the perianal skin.

## Epidemiology

Anal fistulas and abscesses are twice as common in men as in women. Most occur between the ages of 20 and 40 years. Twenty-eight percent of patients with Crohn's disease develop perianal fistulas.

## Patients at risk

Patients with Crohn's disease, persons practicing receptive anal intercourse, prior radiation in the perianal region, prior anal surgery, hematologic malignancies, or prior anal trauma.

## Symptoms

Drainage of pus, anal irritation, pain with defecation, pruritus ani, bleeding, and the sensation of a swelling or an opening near the anus.

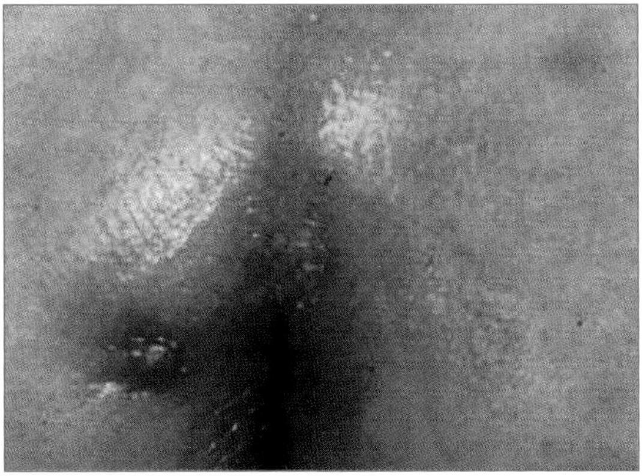

**Figure 1.** A perianal opening can be clearly visualized as a small papule.

## Diagnosis

Physical examination reveals a small external opening with or without drainage (see **Figure 1**). This may look like a tiny skin lesion. According to Goodsall's rule, an imaginary transverse line should be drawn across the anus, and an external lesion seen anterior to this line opens directly from the anal canal (see **Figures 2** and **3**). If the external opening is detected posterior to this line, the fistula is more complex and tracks laterally around the anus prior to a midline posterior opening. Bidigital palpation with the index finger within the anal canal and thumb exterior to the anal canal may enable identification of the entire fistulous track. The internal opening of the fistula may be detectable using a proctoscope or flexible sigmoidoscope. Magnetic resonance imaging (MRI) and anorectal ultrasound are helpful in identifying the full extent of fistulous tracks. Some patients will require an examination under anesthesia.

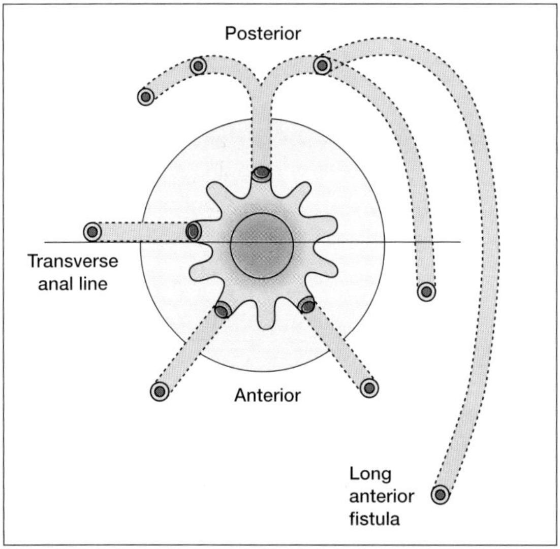


**Figure 2.** Goodsall's rule for finding the internal opening of an anal fistula based on the location of the external opening. When an imaginary line is drawn through the center of the anus, external openings anterior to this line follow a radial (straight) path towards the anal canal. If the external opening is posterior to the line, the fistulous tract will curve and leave the anal canal in the posterior midline.

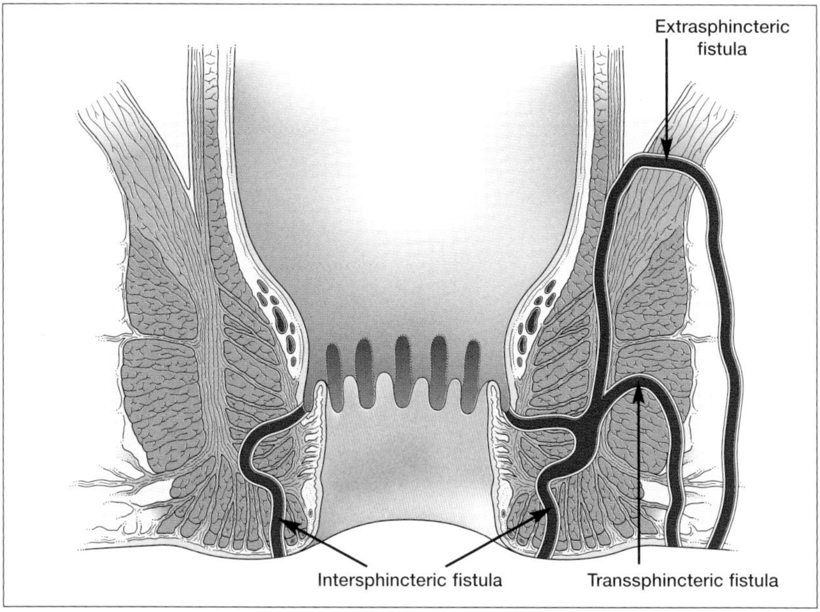


**Figure 3.** Classification of perianal fistulas.

## Treatment

Management of perianal fistulas is generally surgical. For low fistulas (internal opening below the puborectalis muscle), fistulotomy or opening of the fistula track (following the insertion of a probe into the external opening) is utilized. High fistulas (internal opening above the puborectalis muscle) often require closure of the internal opening and performance of an advancement flap. Drainage using a seton may also be performed. Some patients will require a diverting stoma following the repair of a high, complex perianal fistula.

## Clinical pearls

Conservative management and, if possible, avoidance of surgery are recommended in patients with Crohn's disease and perianal fistulas due to difficulty with wound healing and the possible worsening of clinical symptoms as a result of surgery.

# Chapter 3.11

# Proctalgia fugax

## Definition

Episodic, intense anal pain of short duration that is unexplainable following thorough evaluation.

## Epidemiology

Proctalgia fugax occurs in up to 18% of the population of the United States. It is more common in males and individuals who are less than 40 years of age.

## Patients at risk

Persons with irritable bowel syndrome, anxiety, and stress. Proctalgia fugax appears to be more common in patients who are perfectionists or hypochondriacs, and those with a family history of proctalgia fugax.

## Pathophysiology

Proctalgia fugax appears to be due to a sensory dysfunction, with possible hypersensitivity of the internal anal sphincter and rectal musculature. Stressful events appear to precipitate the occurrence of symptoms.

## Symptoms

Proctalgia fugax is defined clinically as the development of sudden, very severe anal pain of very short duration. Pain may last for any length of time from several seconds to 30 minutes. Intensity of the pain ranges from uncomfortable to unbearable. Associated symptoms may include an extreme urge to defecate, diaphoresis, and presyncope.

## Diagnosis

The diagnosis of proctalgia fugax is based on classic symptomatology. Flexible sigmoidoscopy may be performed to rule out other entities.

## Treatment

Careful explanation and reassurance about the condition are critical for treatment. A high-fiber diet, Kegel exercises, and psychotherapy may be beneficial. Inhaled salbutamol may be prescribed for immediate pain relief during episodes. A variety of medical therapies have been attempted including nitroglycerin, amyl nitrate, clonidine, antidepressants, and benzodiazepines. Although success has been reported with these treatments, only a small number of patients were included in the groups studied.

## Clinical pearls

The pain associated with proctalgia fugax is similar to the pain associated with levator ani syndrome. Levator ani syndrome is characterized by episodic anorectal pain and intense spasm of the anal muscles. Patients commonly report difficulty with evacuation. Digital rectal examination reveals marked tenderness of the anal sphincter. Anal tenderness on examination is not a feature of proctalgia fugax.

# Chapter 3.12

# Pruritus ani

## Definition

Itching of the skin around the anus.

## Epidemiology

Pruritus ani is more common in males than females and is the most common anorectal complaint presented to dermatologic specialists.

## Patients at risk

This symptom is usually not associated with the presence of other diseases; however, a large number of conditions can cause pruritus ani (see **Table 1**).

## Pathophysiology

Pruritus ani is more common in individuals who have heightened internal anal sphincter relaxation with rectal distention. This may result in irritation of the perianal region from occult leakage of minute amounts of fecal material from the rectum. Excessive rubbing of the skin results in a decrease in thickness of the fatty skin layer, which exacerbates the problem (see **Figure 1**). Zealous cleansing of the perianal area with alkaline soaps causes contact irritation and dermatitis.

## Symptoms

Itching occurs in the perianal region but may also involve the scrotum or vulva. Symptoms most commonly worsen at night. Little benefit is achieved by scratching the affected area(s) and may worsen the condition.

## Diagnosis

Close examination of the perianal region is required. Scrapings to rule out fungal and yeast infection may be helpful. Anoscopy or flexible sigmoidoscopy has been suggested. Some authors recommend the performance of full colonoscopic evaluation to rule out colorectal pathology such as Crohn's disease. Perianal skin biopsy may be useful in severe cases.

| |
|---|
| Diarrhea, fecal incontinence |
| Hemorrhoids, rectal prolapse |
| Fissures, fistulas |
| Anal scarring, anal stenosis |
| Hidradenitis |
| Malignancy: anal cancer, Bowen's disease, perianal Paget's disease |
| ***Infections*** |
| Fungal: Candidiasis, dermatophytes, *Tinea cruris*, actinomycosis |
| Parasitic: Pinworms, scabies, lice, amoebiasis |
| Bacterial: *Staphylococcus aureus*, tuberculosis |
| Venereal: herpes, gonorrhea, syphilis, condyloma acuminatum |
| ***Local irritants*** |
| Moisture, obesity, excessive perspiration |
| Soaps, hygiene products |
| Toilet paper: perfumed, dyed |
| Underwear: irritating fabrics, detergents |
| Anal creams |
| Dietary: coffee, alcohol, acidic foods, chocolate, nuts, milk |
| Drugs: mineral oil, ascorbic acid, quinidine, colchicine |
| ***Dermatologic diseases*** |
| Psoriasis, eczema |
| Dermatitis (atopic, seborrheic, dermatomyositis) |
| Pemphigus |
| ***Psychogenic*** |
| Anxiety, excessive washing or rubbing of the anal area |
| Autoeroticism |
| ***Systemic disorders*** |
| Diabetes |
| Hyperoxaluria, systemic lupus erythematosus |
| Liver disease |

**Table 1.** Causes of pruritus ani.

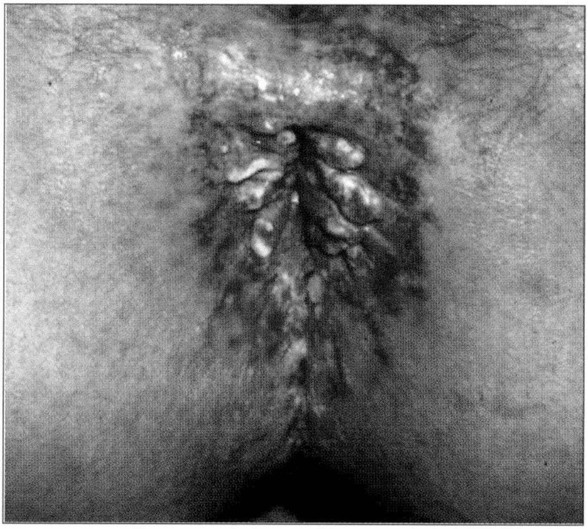

**Figure 1.** Lichenification of the perianal skin due to recurrent pruritus ani.

## Treatment

Explanation and reassurance are required to assist with therapy. Dietary management may be beneficial with temporary elimination of the aforementioned dietary components. Fiber and other bulking agents may also be beneficial. Anal hygiene in the form of cleansing of the perianal region with warm water after each bowel movement is suggested but minimal usage of soap is encouraged. Moistened alcohol free skin wipes that do not contain perfume or witch hazel may be beneficial. Local anesthetic skin ointments are beneficial on an as-needed basis. Chronic therapy with lubricating agents such as Balneol and Tucks may be effective for refractory cases. Colloidal oatmeal-containing baths may also provide relief. Hydrocortisone containing ointments can be used on a temporary basis (less than 3 months).

## Clinical pearls

Pruritus ani is an extremely common complaint. It is often present in patients who practice excessive anal hygiene, particularly following a bowel movement. In our clinic, patients are advised to carry skin wipes in small containers for use after bowel movements; many patients say this is useful. Some authors have stated that more than 90% of patients who follow the above mentioned treatments develop marked improvement in their condition. Refractory patients should be referred to a dermatologist.

# Chapter 3.13

# Radiation proctopathy

## Definition

Acute or chronic injury to the rectum (and/or anus) in patients who have received pelvic irradiation.

## Epidemiology

### Males

There are 180,000 new cases of prostate cancer annually in the United States. Approximately one-third receives radiation therapy.

### Females

There are 36,000 new cases of uterine cancer and 12,000 cases of cervical cancer annually in the United States. Approximately one-third receives radiation therapy.

Symptoms of acute proctopathy occur in up to 30% of radiation therapy patients. Chronic gastrointestinal symptoms are common (estimates vary from 5%–47%).

## Patients at risk

Male and female patients undergoing pelvic radiation therapy.

## Pathophysiology

### Acute radiation proctopathy

Epithelial and vascular endothelial cells develop injury following radiation exposure. Symptoms occur during and up to 6 weeks after completion of a course of radiation therapy.

### Chronic radiation proctopathy

Progressive vascular injury and mucosal epithelial cell destruction occurs. Mucosal atrophy, fibrosis, and secondary telangiectasia formation develop (see **Figures 1** and **2**). Symptoms generally occur 6–12 months after completion of radiation therapy but may be delayed for up to 20 years. Severe complications include rectal ulcerations, stricture formation (see **Figure 3**), bowel obstruction, fistulization (see **Figure 4**), and secondary cancer formation.

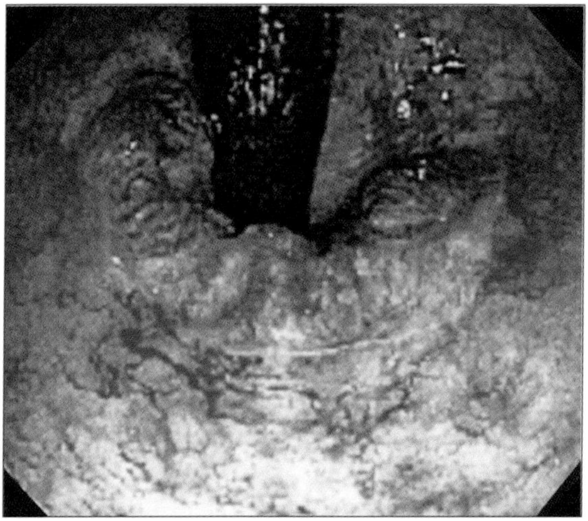

**Figure 1.** Rectal telangiectasia and internal hemorrhoids seen in a patient with radiation therapy.

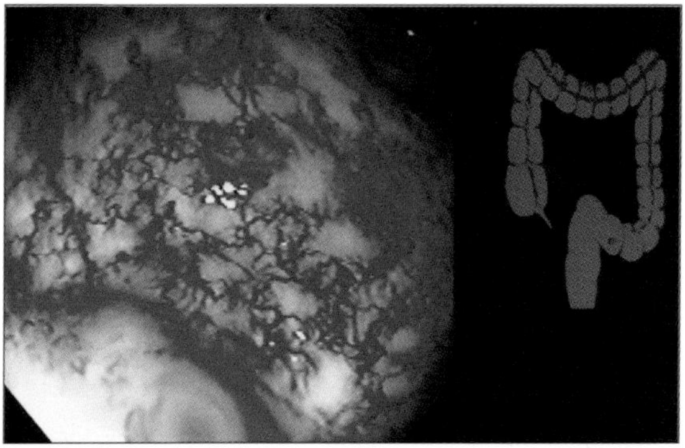

**Figure 2.** Radiation proctopathy characterized by ischemia and telangiectasia formation. No inflammation is present.

## Symptoms

### Acute radiation proctopathy

Diarrhea, straining, and urgency.

### Chronic radiation proctopathy

Rectal bleeding, evacuation difficulty, frequent evacuation, urgency, diarrhea, and fecal incontinence.

## Diagnosis

Flexible sigmoidoscopy to evaluate the affected area. Colonoscopy is indicated for rectal bleeding to rule out other sources.

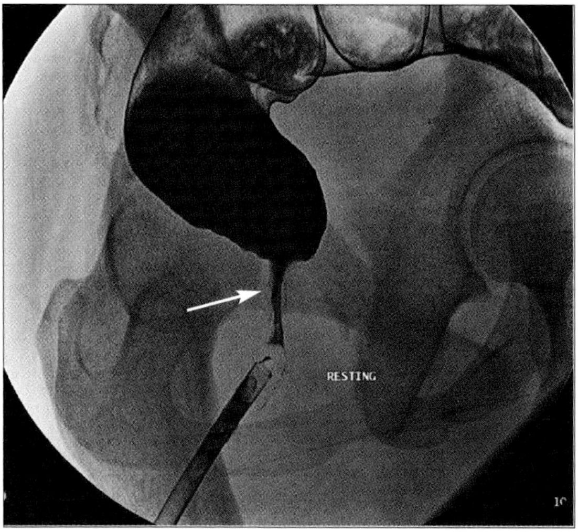


**Figure 3.** Benign anal stricture in a patient with prior radiation therapy (arrow). Tip of catheter present.

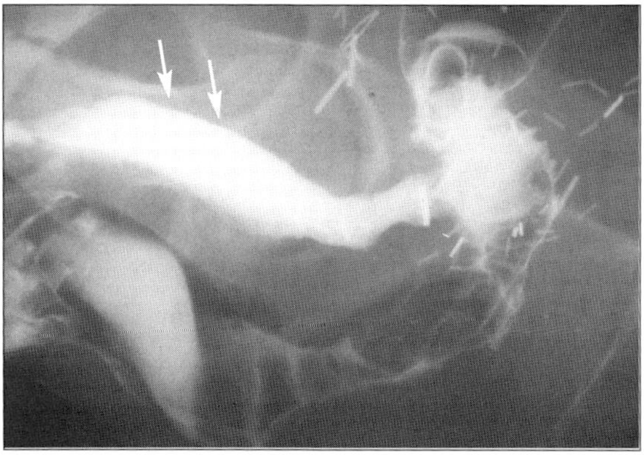

**Figure 4.** Rectovaginal fistula in a patient with prior radiation therapy for cervical cancer. Copious filling of the vagina with barium is seen (arrows).

# Treatment

## Acute radiation proctopathy

Antidiarrheals, a low fiber diet, and change interval of radiation treatment. The radiation oncologist usually institutes these treatments.

## Chronic radiation proctopathy

### *Rectal bleeding*

Endoscopic therapy including laser, argon plasma coagulation, or bipolar electrocautery to obliterate bleeding telangiectasias. Topical formalin application and hyperbaric oxygen therapy may be beneficial. In addition, a role for sucralfate, antioxidants (vitamins C and E), estrogen/progesterone, and corticosteriods has been suggested based on beneficial effects noted in a small number of patients.

### *Other associated symptoms*
Sucralfate, short chain fatty acid enemas, corticosteroids, and 5-ASA compounds may be beneficial. Our group has shown that vitamin A (8000 IU bid) greatly improves these symptoms.

### Surgery
Surgery is reserved for refractory bleeding, bowel obstruction, strictures, and fistulization. Surgery consists of formation of a diverting colostomy or proctectomy. Formation of a colonic J pouch may be performed in younger patients with normal anal sphincter function.

## Clinical pearls

Radiation proctopathies are relatively common disorders, which have received very little attention with regard to development of new treatments. It is anticipated that these conditions will be seen with increasing frequency as the population ages and radiation therapy becomes an acceptable alternative to surgical management for prostate cancer and other pelvic malignancies.

# Chapter 3.14

# Rectal prolapse

## Definition

Displacement of the rectal wall, the anal canal, and the outside of the anus.

## Epidemiology

Rectal prolapse is up to 10-times more common in women than in men. It appears to be most common in multiparous women who are over the age of 50 years.

## Patients at risk

Children with cystic fibrosis, spina bifida, congenital neurologic diseases, Marfan's syndrome, and other congenital mesenchymal diseases. Adults with schistosomiasis, spinal cord disorders, and prolapsing pelvic organs such as the uterus and bladder. In addition, patients with chronic constipation and straining and those with rectal or sigmoid tumors.

## Pathophysiology

Chronic intussusception of the rectal mucosa appears to initiate the condition. A redundant sigmoid colon and decreased external anal sphincter function are aggravating factors. Long-standing rectal prolapse and straining on the toilet result in damage to pelvic nerves, which exacerbates the problem. Overall weakness of the pelvic floor appears to be another important factor. Rectoanal intussusception is the mildest form of rectal prolapse, and occurs when the rectal mucosa prolapses into (but not outside) the anal canal. Prolapse of the mucosa alone may also occur (see **Figure 1**). In the most severe forms of rectal prolapse, all portions of the rectal wall protrude outside of the anus (see **Figure 2**).

## Symptoms

Patients will complain of the sensation of a mass protruding from the rectum upon defecation. A long-standing history of straining can often be elicited. Additional symptoms include rectal bleeding, fecal incontinence, pruritus ani, and rectal pain. In severe cases, inability to reduce the prolapsing rectum and worsening pain may be present. In its most serious form, incarceration of the rectum within and outside of the anal canal may occur with associated ischemia, sepsis, and tissue gangrene.

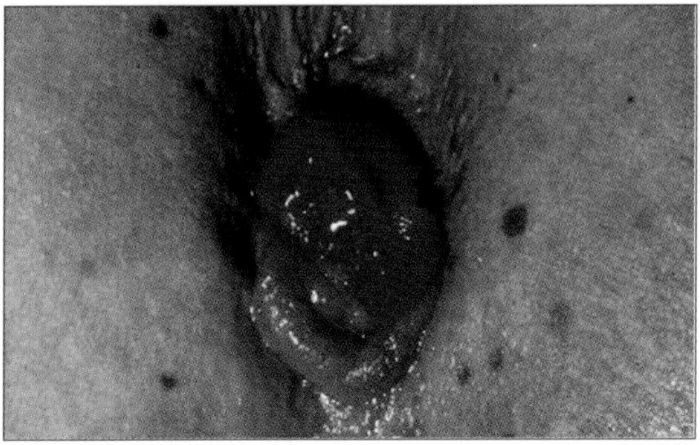

**Figure 1.** Part of the rectal mucosa has prolapsed a few inches from the anal verge.

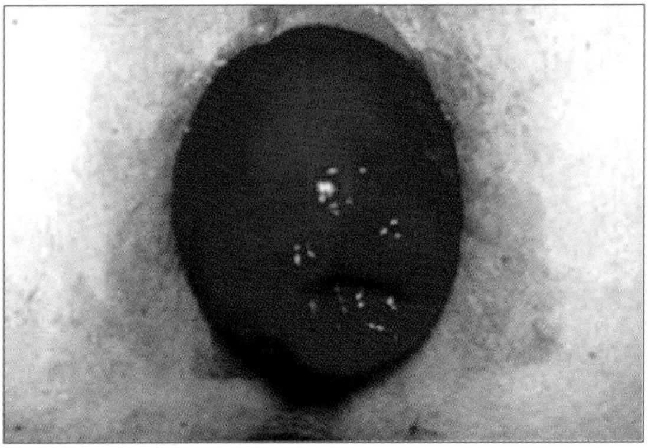

**Figure 2.** Physical examination of an elderly woman demonstrating a complete rectal prolapse.

## Diagnosis

Physical examination with maneuvers to increase intra-abdominal pressure (such as squatting and straining) will demonstrate a rectal prolapse. Presence of prolapsing mucosal folds differentiates rectal prolapse from prolapsing internal hemorrhoids (see **Figure** 3). All patients should have an endoscopic evaluation of the colon to rule out a rectal or sigmoid cancer, which may be present in up to 6% of affected patients. Dynamic proctography will document rectoanal intussusception and rectal prolapse not observed on physical examination (see **Figures** 4 and 5).

## Treatment

### Medical

A complete rectal prolapse is treated with surgery; milder forms may be managed with a high-fiber diet and sitz baths.

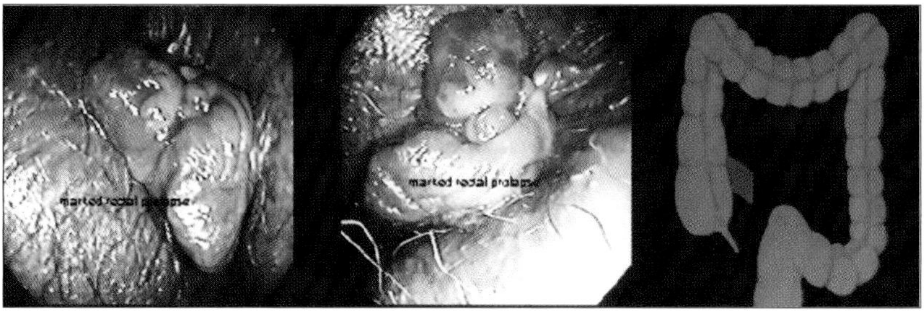


**Figure 3.** Prolapsed internal hemorrhoid.

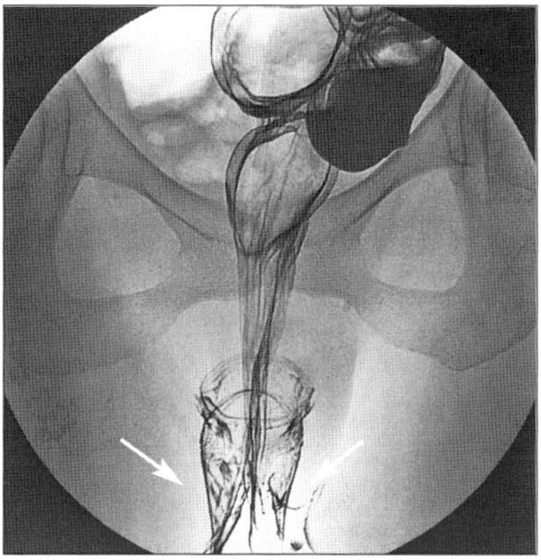

**Figure 4.** Rectal prolapse (arrows) demonstrated on dynamic proctography.

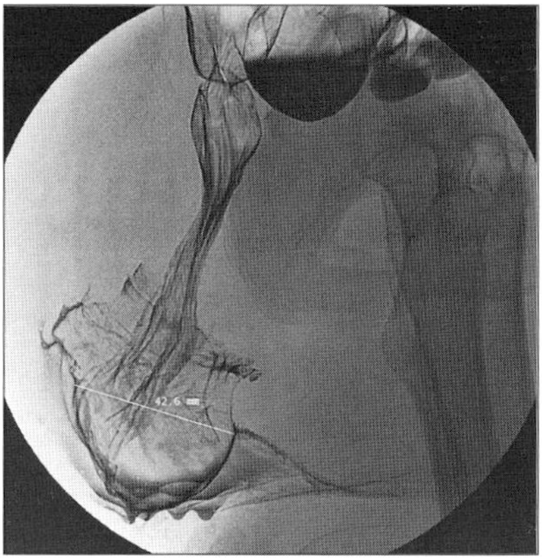

**Figure 5.** Rectal prolapse demonstrated on dynamic proctography on a patient with chronic constipation. Stretching of rectal mucosa noted.

### Surgical

Surgical approaches include anterior resection of the redundant rectum and sigmoid tissue (which can be performed with a transabdominal or perineal approach). Rectopexy (attachment of the rectum to the sacrum with or without mesh) is considered part of surgical management.

## Clinical pearls

Use of pudendal nerve terminal motor latency (PNTML) measurements and anorectal manometry may be beneficial in predicting the functional results of repair of a rectal prolapse. Patients with pudendal nerve damage and/or poor anal sphincter function would be anticipated to have less benefit following surgery for rectal prolapse to improve fecal incontinence.

# Chapter 3.15

# Rectovaginal fistula

## Epidemiology

Rectovaginal fistula is a relatively uncommon condition, seen in some patients with Crohn's disease and rarely has a congenital malformation. Rectovaginal fistula is also a secondary consequence of a variety of injuries to the rectal and vaginal walls.

## Patients at risk

Rectovaginal fistulas most commonly develop as a consequence of obstetric injuries, lacerations, episiotomies, and vaginal lacerations. Other causes include Crohn's disease, damage from pelvic irradiation, anorectal trauma, sigmoid diverticulitis, surgery of the pelvic region including hysterectomy, anal or rectal carcinoma, and foreign body injuries to the rectum.

## Pathophysiology

In Crohn's disease, transmural inflammation of the rectum and anus causes damage to adjacent organs. Associated proteolysis causes tissue destruction and disruption of the normal separation between adjacent organs. Because the anterior wall of the rectum is adjacent to the posterior wall of the vagina, transmural rectal inflammation from Crohn's proctitis results in sinus formation and fistulization (see **Figure 1**). Obstetric injuries from lacerations may extend from the vagina to the rectal wall. Diverticulitis may cause fistulization from the sigmoid colon to the vagina due to diverticular perforation and local extension of inflammation and infection, particularly in patients who have undergone a hysterectomy. Trauma causes either direct penetration between the rectum and vagina or may cause ischemia of either organ, which could lead to fistulization to the other organ during wound healing. Radiation-induced fistulization is generally due to injury to both the rectum and vagina (see **Figure 2**).

## Symptoms

The most common symptoms are the passage of air, feces and/or purulent material from the vagina. Vaginal or rectal bleeding, diarrhea, and fecal incontinence may also occur.

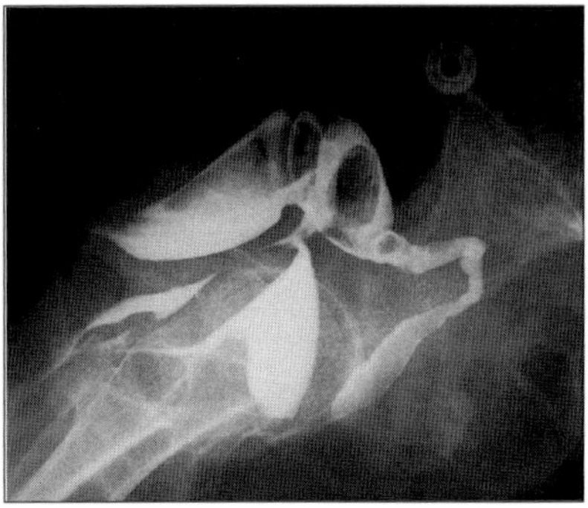

**Figure 1.** Rectovesicular, rectovaginal, and coloenteric fistulas in a patient with Crohn's disease.

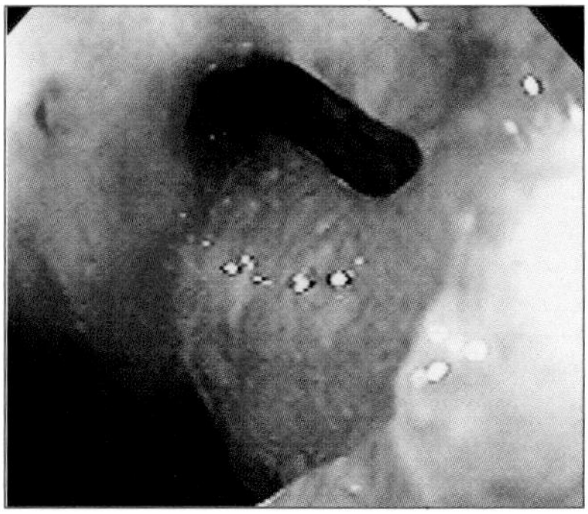

**Figure 2.** Endoscopic view of a rectovaginal fistula in a patient with prior radiation therapy.

## Diagnosis

Physical examination of the anus and vagina occasionally demonstrates a fistula from the anus or the lower portion of the rectum. Identification of the fistula with flexible sigmoidoscopy should be attempted. A barium enema, dynamic proctography, or computed tomography scan may also be useful in visualizing the fistula. If the fistula cannot be identified using these modalities, and the patient has symptoms that are highly suggestive of a rectovaginal fistula, demonstration of the fistula may be achieved by placing a tampon in the vagina followed by instillation of 100 mL of methylene blue into the rectum. Instillation of water or saline into the vagina and placement of a sigmoidoscope in the rectum may also be beneficial: air is injected through the sigmoidoscope, and bubbling of air will be seen in the vagina if a fistula is present.

## Treatment

Rectovaginal fistulas warrant surgical repair. A variety of operations are performed based on the location of the fistula. Techniques for simple fistula repair include transanal repair, transvaginal repair, or endorectal advancement flap placement. Patients with Crohn's disease or radiation-induced rectovaginal fistulas may require a proctectomy. Some patients with radiation injuries have benefited from muscle flap interposition between the two organs, which improves the rate of successful repair.

## Clinical pearls

It is often difficult to identify rectovaginal fistulas in the upper portion of the vagina, particularly in women who have undergone a hysterectomy. In these cases, fistulization occurs at the vaginal cuff. Some of the previously described maneuvers may be required to identify the presence of these fistulas.

# Chapter 3.16

# Solitary rectal ulcer syndrome

## Definition

A disorder characterized by rectal mucosal damage and rectal bleeding with anorectal pain.

## Epidemiology

Solitary rectal ulcer syndrome (SRUS) is seen in individuals who strain during defecation. It has also been associated with rectal prolapse, self-digitization, and spastic anorectal disorders such as nonrelaxing puborectalis syndrome.

## Patients at risk

SRUS is more common in female young adults, and is seen in individuals performing manual disimpaction, persons practicing anal autoeroticism, and victims of rape or sexual abuse.

## Pathophysiology

SRUS appears to be caused by mucosal ischemia and ulceration. It may be triggered by rectal prolapse causing decreased blood flow. Hamartomatous malformation and congenital duplication of rectal mucosa may be factors contributing to its development. Repeated straining in individuals with nonrelaxing puborectalis syndrome may worsen the condition. Histologically, there is replacement of the lamina propria near the ulcer with collagen and muscle fibers of the muscularis mucosa. Inflammatory changes occur at the site of the ulceration.

## Symptoms

The most common symptom of SRUS is rectal bleeding (98%). Constipation, discharge of mucus, tenesmus, and pain in the sacrum or perineum also occur. More than 50% of patients will complain of chronic constipation.

## Diagnosis

Flexible sigmoidoscopy or colonoscopy is utilized to make a diagnosis. Endoscopically, discrete or multiple ulcerations with surrounding erythema and induration may be seen. Other descriptions include a raised erythematous region, polypoid region, or plaque-like regions. Lesions are most commonly present in the anterior rectal wall, generally 7–10 cm proximal to the anal verge. Biopsies show classic histologic findings as described above.

## Treatment

### Lifestyle

Avoidance of straining, discontinuation of rectal digitation, a high-fiber diet.

### Medical

Laxatives and stool softeners may be beneficial. Sucralfate and hydrocortisone enemas have been suggested but are unproven therapies.

### Surgical

Rectopexy before repair of rectal prolapse, insertion of a perianal nylon loop, and myotomy of the puborectalis muscle in cases of nonrelaxing puborectalis syndrome. Colostomy may be indicated in cases of severe rectal bleeding.

## Clinical pearls

SRUS is frequently misdiagnosed and confused with other conditions such as inflammatory bowel disease and rectal masses such as villous adenoma.

# Chapter 3.17

# Ulcerative proctitis

## Definition

A chronic inflammatory bowel disorder only affecting the rectum.

## Epidemiology

The epidemiology of ulcerative proctitis is similar to ulcerative colitis. Approximately 40% of patients with ulcerative colitis only have manifestations of the disease in the rectum or rectosigmoid colon. Ulcerative colitis occurs throughout the world but is most common in the white population of the United States. Ulcerative colitis is especially common in Jews of Eastern European origin. A number of factors have been identified that appear to predispose to the condition: the ethnic and racial distribution of ulcerative colitis suggests a genetic component of the disorder; environmental factors also play a role. For example, prior appendectomy protects against ulcerative colitis. Additionally, ulcerative colitis is more common in former tobacco smokers and nonsmokers than in current tobacco users.

## Pathophysiology

The mechanism for the development of ulcerative proctitis is similar to that of ulcerative colitis. It is an autoimmune condition characterized by the presence of antibodies to various components of the gastrointestinal mucosa. Cytotoxic T-cell function appears to be enhanced, most likely in response to elevated inflammatory cytokines. Activation of monocytes and T-cells causes increased secretion of a variety of cytokines including tumor necrosis factor-α, interleukin-1, and interleukin-6.

Endoscopically, the disease is characterized by the presence of mucosal inflammation beginning at the anal verge and extending without interruption in a proximal fashion. This is in contrast to Crohn's disease, which commonly spares the rectum and is characterized by "skip areas" of normal mucosa between inflamed portions of the bowel. Depending on the severity of the inflammation, erythema, edema, granularity, friable hemorrhagic mucosa, loss of normal vascular pattern, punctate ulcerations, larger deep ulcerations, and advanced disease with

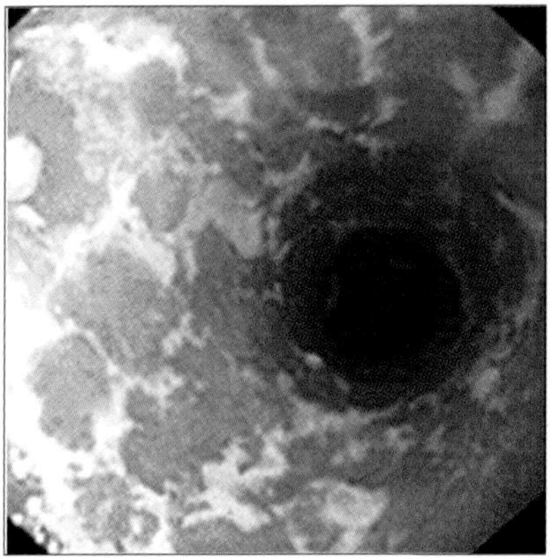

**Figure 1.** Endoscopic view of moderate colitis demonstrating ulceration, exudates, and loss of vascular pattern of mucosa.

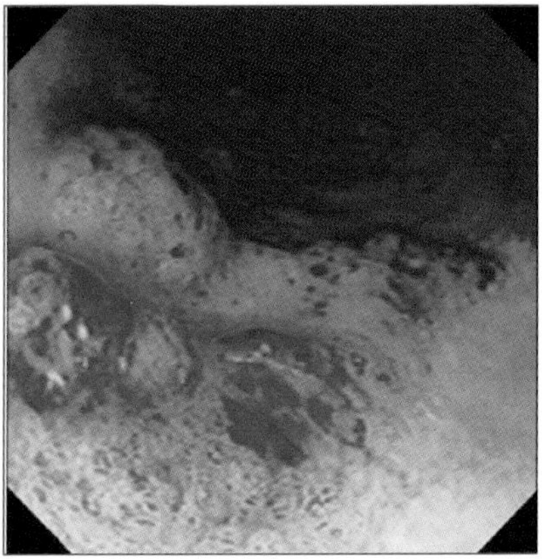

**Figure 2.** Typical endoscopic appearance of a dysplasia-associated lesion or mass (DALM) in ulcerative colitis.

complete denuding of the mucosa may be seen (see **Figure 1**). Long-standing ulcerative colitis may be characterized by chronic stricture formation; however, the presence of a stricture in a patient with ulcerative colitis should raise concern that a secondary carcinoma may have developed.

Microscopically, mucosal inflammation is seen with edema and hemorrhage in the lamina propria. Mucosal infiltration with a variety of inflammatory cells produces cryptitis and crypt abscess formation. Long-standing ulcerative colitis may result in the development of dysplasia and secondary carcinoma (see **Figure 2**); however, this appears to be less common in patients with proctitis alone.

## Symptoms

The most common symptoms of ulcerative colitis are diarrhea and rectal bleeding. Patients with ulcerative proctitis and left-sided ulcerative colitis often have symptoms of rectal urgency, incomplete evacuation, tenesmus, and, occasionally, fecal incontinence. More severe disease is characterized by systemic symptoms including fever, weight loss, and signs and symptoms of anemia.

## Diagnosis

Sigmoidoscopy is generally utilized to make the initial diagnosis of ulcerative colitis and ulcerative proctitis. Careful description of the findings on sigmoidoscopy is recommended to indicate the endoscopic severity of the disease. Biopsies are obtained to diagnose ulcerative colitis and to rule out other forms of colitis including infectious colitis, ischemic colitis, pseudomembranous colitis, and nonsteroidal anti-inflammatory drug-induced colitis. Because rectal bleeding and changing bowel habits may indicate the presence of other diseases, eg, colonic malignancy. Evaluation of the entire colon with a colonoscopy may be required if typical symptoms of colitis are not revealed on sigmoidoscopy. Colonoscopy is also used to determine the extent of colonic involvement and endoscopic severity of the disease.

# Treatment

## Medical

Mild to moderate disease is initially treated with 5-ASA-containing agents administered either by mouth or rectally in the form of a suppository or enema. These drugs are also used for maintenance therapy of the disease. More severe cases are treated acutely with corticosteroids given either parenterally, orally, or into the rectum. Patients requiring repeated courses of corticosteroid treatment are started on immune-modulating agents (so-called steroid-sparing drugs) such as azathioprine and 6-mercaptopurine.

Typical doses for treatment are as follows:

- Acute colitis (severe): prednisone 40–60 mg/day with dose tapering following relief of symptoms. Hospitalized patients are treated with methylprednisolone 40 mg/day by continuous intravenous (IV) drip, or 15 mg IV piggyback (IVBP) four times per day.
- Acute colitis (mild to moderate) and maintenance therapy: oral mesalamine 2.4–4 g/day. A variety of forms of mesalamine are available on the market. These vary in their release properties and the vehicle that is utilized to prevent the destruction of mesalamine prior to delivery to the appropriate inflamed portions of the gastrointestinal tract. Mesalamine suppositories (500 mg dose) are administered once or twice today. Mesalamine retention enemas are given as a single 4 g (60 mL) dose that is retained for 8 hours at night. Recommended doses of azathioprine and 6-mercaptopurine (which are generally reserved for maintenance therapy in patients requiring repeated corticosteroid treatment) are 2.5 mg/kg/day and 1.5 mg/kg/day, respectively.

## Surgical

Surgery is indicated for acute disease that is refractory to IV corticosteroid therapy (or cyclosporine in some centers), or complicated by perforation or toxic megacolon. Surgery is also indicated for chronic poorly controlled disease, and the secondary development of cancer, precancerous lesions, or dysplasia.

Total proctocolectomy is the surgical treatment of choice for ulcerative colitis. In elderly patients, or patients who are unable to undergo further surgery, a permanent Brook ileostomy is performed. In younger patients with intact anal sphincter functions an ileoanal anastomosis and creation of an ileal pouch (also known as a J pouch) will be performed. Surgeries are most commonly recommended for patients with pancolitis (involving the entire colon). It is very uncommon for patients with ulcerative proctitis alone to require surgical therapy.

## Clinical pearls

Recent studies, including meta-analyses of the medical literature, indicate that therapy with topical mesalamine is more effective than oral mesalamine in the treatment of acute ulcerative proctitis and for maintenance therapy of the disease.

Since the risk of colon cancer increases dramatically in patients who have had ulcerative colitis for more than 10 years, regular surveillance colonoscopy with multiple mucosal biopsies throughout the colon is performed. Surveillance colonoscopy is recommended annually for those patients who have had ulcerative colitis for 10 years or who have pancolitis, and every 2–3 years in patients with ulcerative proctitis.

# Chapter 4

# Neoplasms of the anus

# Chapter 4.1

# Anal carcinoma

## Tumor subtypes

### Cloacal

Cloacal tumors arise from the transitional epithelium lined zone separating the rectum from the squamous-lined portion of the anal canal proximal to the dentate line.

### Squamous cell

Squamous cell tumors arise from the squamous epithelium in the anal canal.

### Perianal skin and anal margin tumors

These tumors arise from keratinized, hair-bearing skin near the entrance of the anal canal (see **Figure 1**).

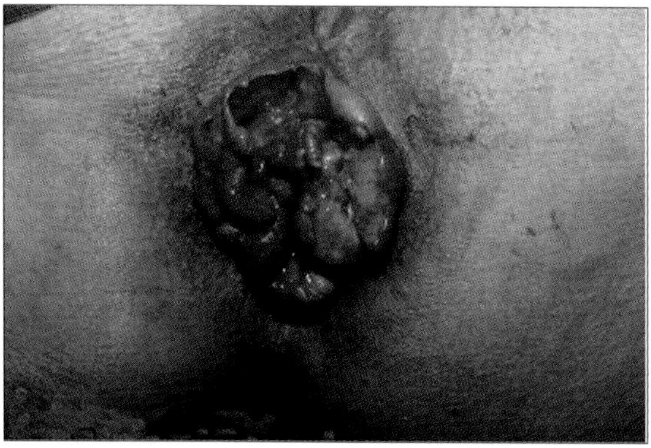

**Figure 1.** A large anal tumor with ulcerating components is seen on external examination in this elderly female.

## Epidemiology

The average age of presentation is 57 years. Anal canal tumors are more common in women (60%), whereas perianal skin and anal margin tumors are more common in men (80%).

## Patients at risk

Homosexual men; people who practice receptive anal intercourse; people infected with HIV or human papillomavirus (HPV); people with anal condylomata, cervical cancer, chronic anal fistula, a prior history of syphilis, a prior infection with herpes simplex virus type II, or perianal Crohn's disease; people who have undergone anal irradiation or renal transplantation; and people who smoke.

## Symptoms

The most common symptoms are rectal bleeding and pain in the anorectal region; however, 75% of patients are asymptomatic. Pruritus ani, a sensation of fullness or a lump in the anal region, anal discharge, a change in bowel habits, or pain in the pelvic region may occur.

## Pathophysiology

A strong relationship exists between anal and genital HPV infection and the development of anal carcinoma. It is assumed that previous infection with HPV places individuals at risk for the condition. Environmental factors such as cigarette smoking and exposure to other sexually transmitted diseases appear to be important variables. Finally, immunosuppression appears to further promote carcinogenesis.

## Diagnosis

Visual inspection is performed initially and may include digital rectal exam, anoscopy, sigmoidoscopy, or a barium study (see **Figures 2** and **3**). Anesthesia is often required for full evaluation. Diagnosis is made by biopsy of the lesion.

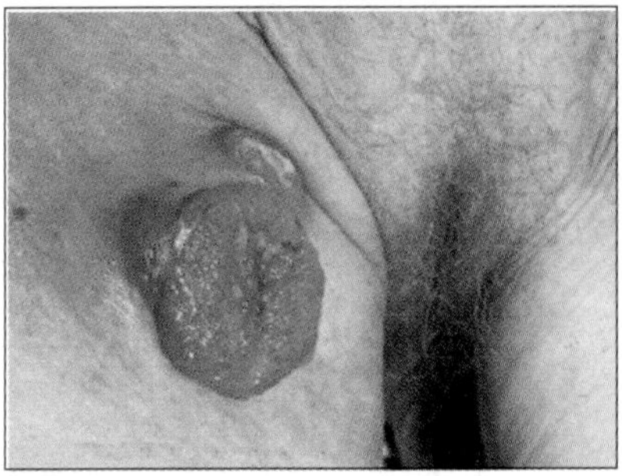

**Figure 2.** Anal carcinoma with secondary inguinal lymph node deposit.

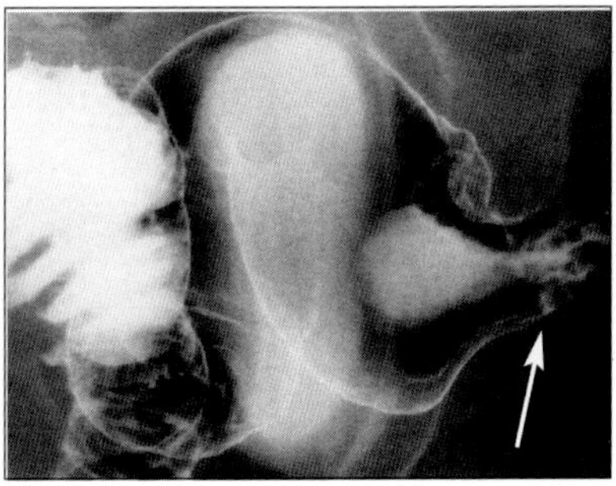

**Figure 3.** Barium study demonstrates irregular appearance of lesion (arrow).

# Treatment

### Surgical

If the lesion is small, involving only the mucosa and submucosa, a wide local excision is performed. Large, advanced lesions require an abdominal–perineal resection and colostomy formation.

### Combination radiation and chemotherapy (the Nigro protocol)

External beam radiation (30 Gy) is administered over a 3-week period. Concomitant 5-fluorouracil is administered continuously for the first 4 days and again on days 29–32. Mitomycin-C is also given on the first day of treatment. An 85% success rate is expected, and most patients undergoing the Nigro protocol will not require an abdominal–perineal resection or colostomy.

# Clinical pearls

Patients undergoing the Nigro protocol should receive frequent follow-up examinations and biopsies of the anorectal region to evaluate for recurrence. Occasionally, carcinoma of the anus will be discovered in a hemorrhoidectomy specimen. These patients also require surveillance. Some have suggested that patients with perianal or genital condyloma and other forms of HPV infection should undergo routine surveillance for anal carcinoma.

# Chapter 4.2

# Other anal malignancies

## Anal adenocarcinoma

### Symptoms

The most common symptoms are anal pain, bleeding, sensation of a mass, and fistula drainage.

### Pathophysiology

This is a rare tumor that arises from anal glandular tissue. It is often seen developing in anorectal fistulas.

### Diagnosis

Physical examination, anoscopy, and/or flexible sigmoidoscopy.

### Treatment

Treatment is usually surgical, the most common procedure being abdominoperineal resection.

### Prognosis

The recurrence rate after surgery is very high (54%), and estimated mean survival is between 2–3 years. Due to this high rate of recurrence, some investigators have recommended preoperative chemotherapy and radiation therapy.

## Basal cell carcinoma of the perianal region

### Epidemiology

This is a rare location for basal cell carcinoma and is stated to represent less than 0.1% of all cases of anorectal tumors. It is more common in men and generally occurs after the age of 50 years.

### Symptoms

The most common symptoms are bleeding, ulceration, or a lump-like sensation in the perianal region.

### Pathophysiology

This tumor arises from the basal cells of the perianal skin.

### Diagnosis
This tumor classically appears as an exophytic lesion (a neoplasm or lesion that grows outward from an epithelial surface) with rolled edges and a central ulceration.

### Treatment
These lesions are treated with local incision, sometimes in combination with radiation therapy.

### Prognosis
Local recurrences occur in 29% of patients and the 5-year survival rate is 73%.

## Bowen's disease

### Epidemiology
This is a rare intraepidermal squamous cell carcinoma.

### Pathophysiology
Bowen's disease appears to be a marker for the development of other carcinomas including bronchogenic carcinoma, genitourinary tumors, and gastrointestinal adenocarcinoma.

### Diagnosis
It is a slow-growing tumor that is rarely invasive.

### Treatment
The lesion is treated with local wide incision.

## Malignant melanoma

### Epidemiology
This is a rare tumor that accounts for 0.5%–1% of all anal cancers, and 0.2%–1.6% of all melanomas. Anal melanoma appears to be more than twice as common in women as in men.

### Pathophysiology
This tumor arises from melanocytes in the squamous mucosa of the anal canal and possibly the lower rectum.

### Symptoms
The most common symptoms are pain, a lump like sensation in the anal region, constipation and evacuation difficulty, and change in bowel habits. Anorectal bleeding may also occur.

### Diagnostic testing

Physical examination with visualization of the external perianal region is often sufficient to identify the lesion. Lesions higher in the anal canal or in the lower rectum will be seen on flexible sigmoidoscopy or anoscopy.

### Treatment

Surgical resection is required. It appears that local resection has the same overall prognosis as radical resection. Adjuvant chemotherapy and radiation therapy have not been proven to be beneficial.

### Prognosis

Very poor; 5-year survival has been estimated to be between 0%–5%.

## Perianal Paget's disease

### Epidemiology

This is a rare disorder that resembles Paget's disease of the breast. Average age at diagnosis is approximately 60 years.

### Symptoms

Rectal bleeding, discharge, pruritus ani, and pain.

### Pathophysiology

Perianal Paget's disease is characterized histologically as a dermatosis with multiple large vascular cells present within the epithelium. Histologically, the cells resemble those of Bowen's disease and are differentiated by positive periodic acid-Schiff staining. Perianal Paget's disease is closely associated with the presence of carcinoma of the anus and rectum.

### Diagnosis

Physical examination reveals an erythematous plaque with crusting and scaling.

### Treatment

Treatment may include topical retinoid therapy, local surgical resection, and abdominoperineal resection depending on the stage of the disease.

### Prognosis

The majority (<75%) of patients with perianal Paget's disease have an adjacent anal carcinoma. Five-year survival has been estimated at about 50%.

# Chapter 5

# Neoplasms of the rectum

# Chapter 5.1

# Rectal carcinoma

## Epidemiology

Rectal carcinoma occurs most commonly in patients between 50 and 70 years of age. It is equally common in males and females.

## Patients at risk

Patients with sporadic adenomatous colonic polyps, familial polyposis coli, long-standing ulcerative colitis, a family history of colorectal polyps and colorectal cancers, long-standing Crohn's colitis, or presence of a ureteral diversion colostomy. Other risks include prior radiation therapy, long-standing use of stimulant laxatives, and cholecystectomy.

## Pathophysiology

Mutations of oncogenes – genes that transform normal cells into abnormally proliferating cells – are commonly seen in colorectal cancers and large adenomas. Abnormalities in a variety of tumor suppressor genes including *DCC* (deleted in colon cancer), *APC* (familial adenomatous polyposis coli gene), *MSH2*, *MLH1*, *PMS1*, *PMS2*, and *MSH6* (hereditary nonpolyposis colorectal cancer genes) have been identified. Patients with APC, an autosomal dominant disease defined by the presence of at least 100 adenomatous polyps within the colon, develop colorectal cancers by the age of 40 years (see **Figure 1**).

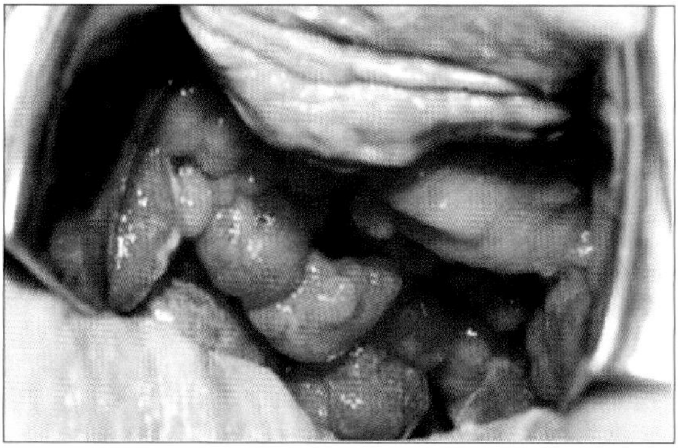

**Figure 1.** A 24-year-old woman with familial adenomatous polyposis coli (APC) has numerous polyps in the rectum, some of which have prolapsed, as seen on sigmoidoscopy.

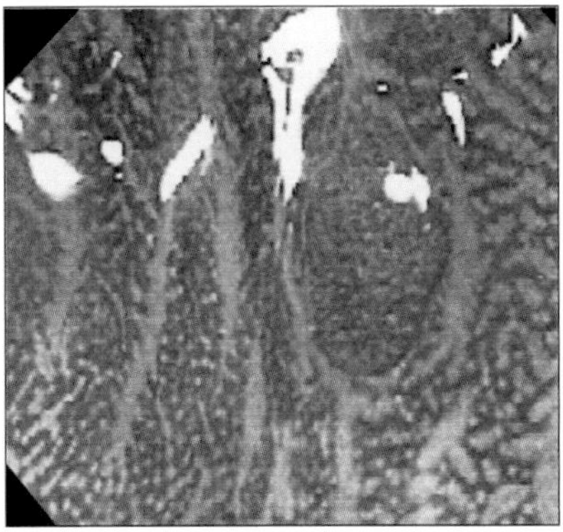

**Figure 2.** Magnified view of colon mucosa stained with methylene blue demonstrating an aberrant crypt focus, a possible precursor of adenomatous tissue (photo courtesy of Dr Gregory Cohen).

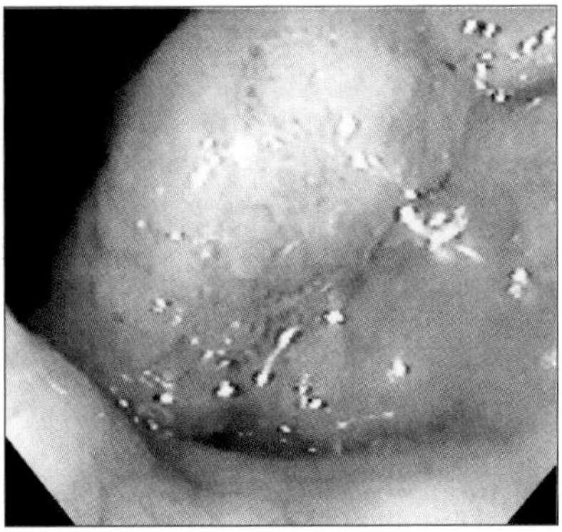

**Figure 3.** Sessile rectal polyp determined to contain invasive adenocarcinoma.

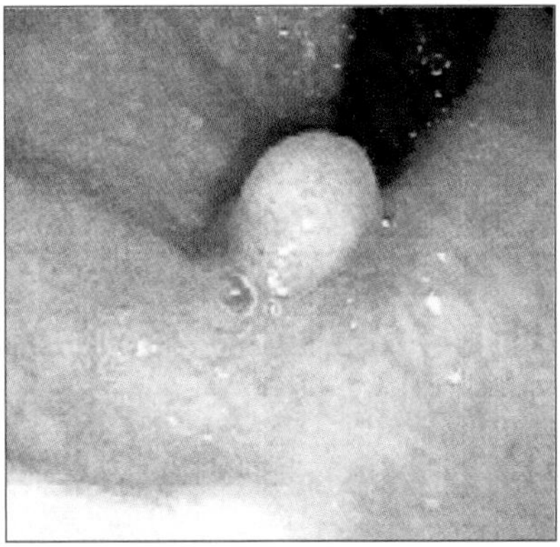

**Figure 4.** A sessile polyp near the dentate line seen on retroflexion during colonoscopy.

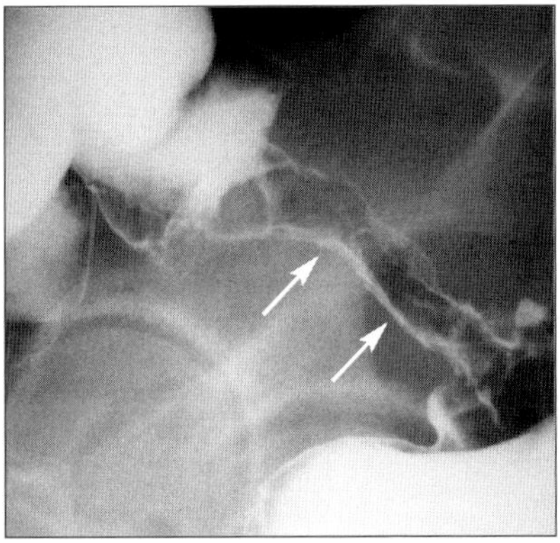

**Figure 5.** Advanced rectal carcinoma. Lateral view on barium study shows large "apple core" lesion (arrows).

The mutated *APC* gene, located on chromosome five, has been isolated in this patient group. Colorectal cancers generally begin as aberrant crypt foci and develop into adenomatous polyps (see **Figures 2–4**). Dysplasia within these lesions becomes more frequent as the size of the polyps increases.

Tubulovillous and villous adenomatous polyps are more likely to have associated dysplasia or intramucosal carcinoma than tubular adenomas. The prevalence of colonic adenomas appears to be about 25% in persons over the age of 50 years.

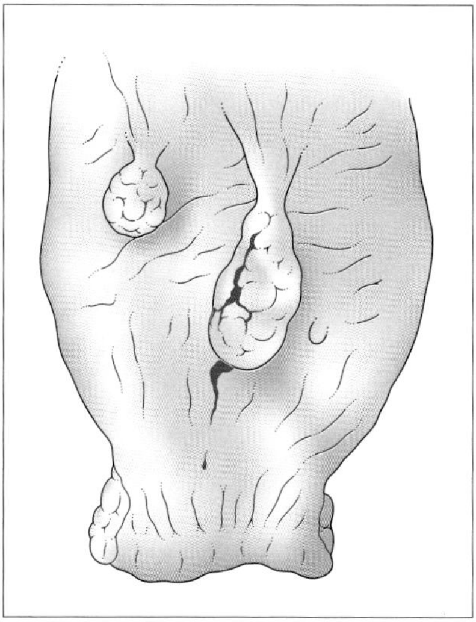

**Figure 6.** Pedunculated rectal polyps as seen on endoscopy.

Environmental factors clearly play a role in the development of colorectal polyps and cancer. The prevalence of colorectal cancer in industrialized countries ranges from 10–35 per 100,000 people, while prevalence in Third World countries ranges from 0.2–10 per 100,000 people. People from countries with a low prevalence of colorectal carcinoma who move to countries with a high prevalence, eg, Japanese people who have moved to Hawaii, have a much higher prevalence of colorectal cancer than natives of the low prevalence population. High-fat, low fiber diets have been implicated in the increased incidence of colorectal cancer. Obesity and decreased activity also appear to play a role.

## Symptoms

Approximately 50% of rectal cancers are asymptomatic at the time of diagnosis. More advanced lesions present with rectal bleeding, change in bowel habits, constipation, obstipation, tenesmus, and passage of thin, narrow stools (see **Figure 5**). Very advanced lesions may present with the signs and symptoms of iron deficiency anemia, rectal pain, rectal obstruction, weight loss and malaise, colonic perforation, or the signs and symptoms of metastatic disease.

## Diagnosis

Digital rectal examination may result in palpation of the lesion (generally if it is within 10 cm of the anal verge). Testing of the stool may reveal the presence of occult blood. Proctoscopy, flexible sigmoidoscopy, or endoscopy is used to visualize the lesion and to obtain biopsies (see **Figure 6**). Full colonoscopy is utilized to evaluate for synchronous colorectal neoplasms.

## Treatment

In lesions that are restricted to the mucosa, transanal resection with excision of surrounding normal mucosa may be utilized. Endoscopic mucosal resection has recently been advocated as an alternative treatment for rectal cancer that only involves the mucosa (see **Figure 7**). Larger, more advanced lesions are treated surgically with a low anterior resection or an abdominoperineal resection (see **Surgery for rectal cancer**). Preoperative or postoperative radiation therapy and chemotherapy are indicated with curative intent for stage II and III cancer, and are indicated for palliation in patients with stage IV disease (see **Staging of rectal cancer**).

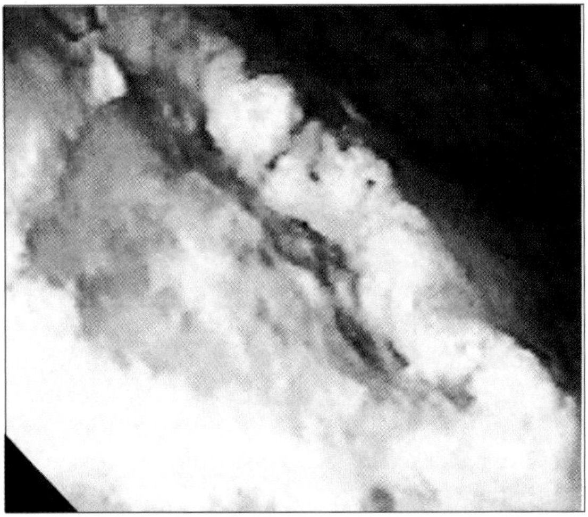

**Figure 7.** Sessile rectal polyp determined to contain invasive adenocarcinoma as seen after endoscopic mucosal resection (photo courtesy of Dr Charles Dye).

## Clinical pearls

Regular screening for colorectal neoplasms with full colonic evaluation using colonoscopy has recently been approved in the United States for patients of 50 years or older. New screening methods, including the use of stool-based molecular tests and radiographic methods such as computed tomography colonography, are undergoing investigation.

# Chapter 5.2

# Staging of rectal cancer

## Modified Dukes' classification

The purpose of staging colorectal cancers is to determine appropriate therapies for individual patients and to establish the prognosis for each case. Specifically, staging helps to determine whether adjuvant chemotherapy and radiation therapy should be utilized in an attempt to cure the disease. The Dukes' classification system was originally established in the 1930s (see **Table 1**). It is based on the depth of tumor penetration and the presence or absence of lymph node involvement. The 5-year survival following surgery in patients who were deemed potentially curable is listed with each stage (for colon and rectal cancer).

## TNM classification

The American Joint Committee for cancer staging and end results developed this system as an alternative to the Dukes' classification system. The TNM system (T: tumor; N: nodes; M: metastases) analyzes in detail the degree of local and regional spread of the tumor (see **Figure 1**).

### Stage 0

Carcinoma *in situ*.

### Stage I

Tumor extends into the submucosa (T1, N0, M0).

Tumor extends to and invades the muscularis propria (T2, N0, M0).

### Stage II

Tumor extends to and invades the subserosa, nonperitonealized pericolonic tissue, or perirectal tissue (T3, N0, M0).

Tumor extends to and perforates the visceral peritoneum or directly invades nearby organs and other structures (T4, N0, M0).

| Classification | Stage A | Stage B1 | Stage B2 | Stage C1 | Stage C2 | Stage D |
|---|---|---|---|---|---|---|
| Disease progression | 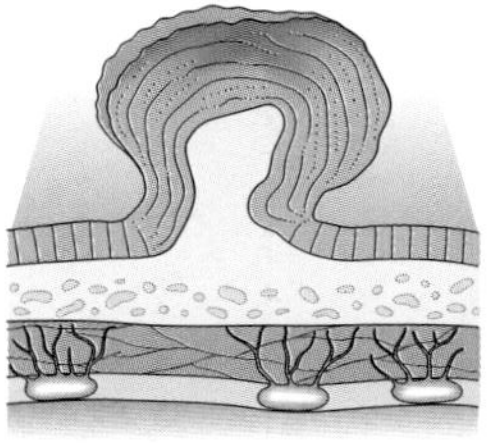 | 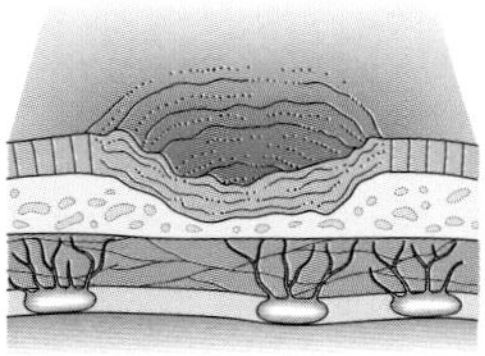 | | 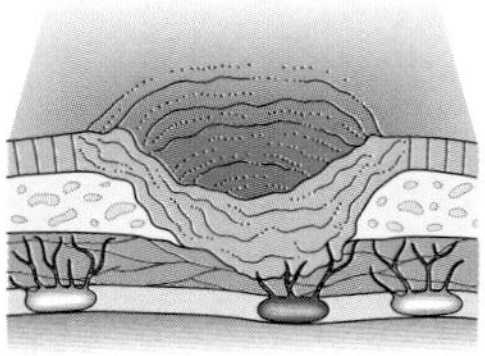 | | 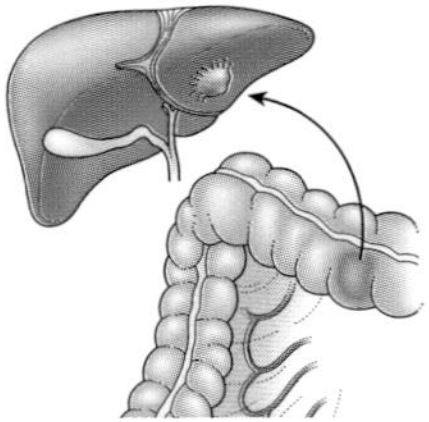 |
| | Tumor is restricted to the mucosa only | Tumor invades into the muscularis propria | Tumor invades through the muscularis propria and serosa | Tumor invades the muscularis propria and is found in regional lymph nodes | Tumor invades the muscularis propria (and extends into the serosa) and is found in regional lymph nodes | Tumor has metastasized to distant organs such as liver, lungs, and bone |
| Estimated 5-year survival | 90% | 80% | 60% | 40% | 40% | 0% |

**Table 1.** Dukes' classification of adenocarcinoma of the colon or rectum.

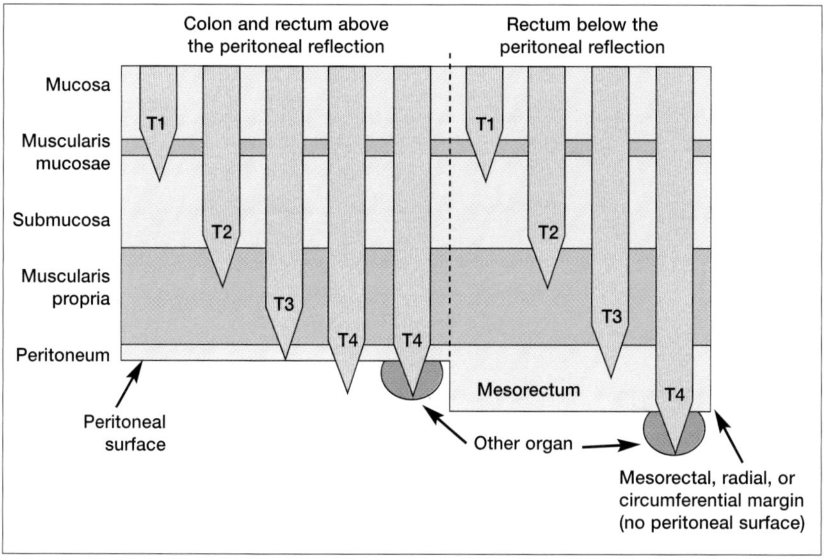


**Figure 1.** TNM staging of colorectal carcinoma.

## Stage III

This stage is defined by nodal involvement. Therefore, any tumor with associated lymph node metastasis is a stage III tumor. Tumor perforates the bowel wall and metastasizes to regional lymph nodes.

N1: 1–3 pericolonic or perirectal lymph nodes.

N2: 4 or more pericolonic or perirectal lymph nodes.

N3: Involvement of lymph nodes along any named vascular structure.

## Stage IV

Tumor has metastasized to distant organs such as the liver, lungs, and bone.

Microscopic grading of the degree of differentiation of the tumor is also used to determine prognosis. Pathologic grading is as follows:

- Grade 1 (well differentiated) – epithelial proliferation.
- Grade 2 (moderately differentiated) – glandular pattern present but more crowded.
- Grade 3 (poorly differentiated) – anaplastic cells, frequent mitosis.
- Grade 4 (mucinous tumors) – more than 50% of tumor volume is occupied by mucin.

# Chapter 5.3

# Surgery for rectal cancer

## General information

Several different surgical techniques are employed for rectal cancer depending on the location and the tumor stage. The primary goal of surgery is the complete removal of the tumor. When possible, surgical techniques are also employed that result in the preservation of continence. Recent advances in surgical therapy, particularly with the improvement of low anterior resections with double-stapling devices, have allowed more patients to avoid the requirement of a permanent ostomy after surgery for rectal cancer.

## Abdominoperineal resection

Abdominoperineal resection (APR) is performed when there is an inadequate distal margin of the rectum (<2 cm); when there is a large, bulky pelvic tumor present; and when there is evidence of local tumor extension beyond the rectum. This surgery involves an *en-bloc* dissection of the retroperitoneum between the ureters, resulting in removal of the anus, rectum, and distal sigmoid colon. Complete removal of the rectal mesentery (mesorectum) with lymph node removal (total mesorectal excision) is also usually performed (see **Figure 1**). A permanent sigmoid colostomy is constructed.

## Low anterior resection

This surgery is performed when there is at least a 2-cm margin of normal tissue distal to the tumor. The development of the double-stapling technique has allowed an increased number of patients with more distal rectal tumors to undergo low anterior resections and avoid an APR. Coloanal anastomosis and the occasional construction of colonic J pouches are also new surgical techniques allowing preservation of the anal sphincters and avoidance of APR. Complete mesorectal excision has also been advocated in conjunction with low anterior resections and has been repeatedly demonstrated to reduce the local recurrence rate of rectal cancers.

## Transanal resection

This surgery is performed on tumors that are ≤4 cm in diameter and involve the mucosa only (Stage A, Dukes' classification). These tumors should be palpable and

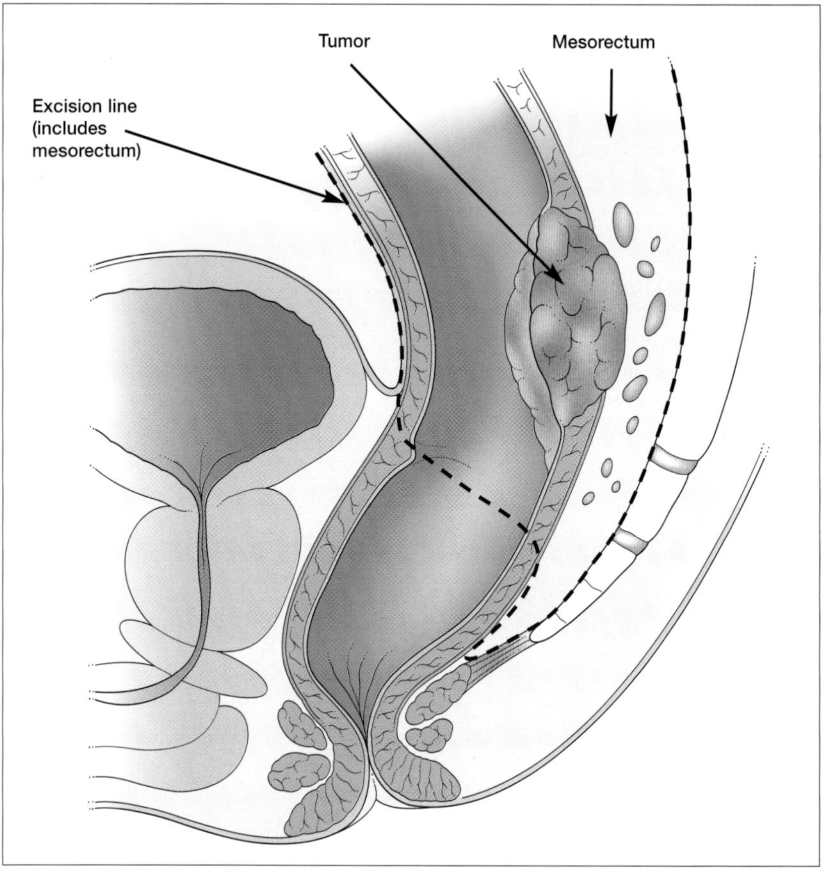


**Figure 1.** The area removed during mesorectal resection.

freely mobile by digital rectal examination. Tumors should be <9 cm from the anal verge and no lymph nodes should be detected on endoscopic ultrasound. The procedure is performed using a proctoscope or with anal dilatation and retractor insertion. Removal of a margin (of about 1 cm) of normal mucosa around the tumor with a full thickness resection of the rectal wall is performed.

## Additional comments

The use of endoscopic mucosal resection has been advocated by some as an alternative to transanal resection for small rectal tumors. Since this technique involves resection of the mucosa only, I would only advocate this procedure for rectal cancer in patients who are extremely high-risk transanal resection patients.

# Chapter 5.4

# Medical therapy for rectal cancer

Local recurrence after resection for rectal cancer is common (average 30% local recurrence rate). Patients with TNM stage II (Dukes' B2) rectal cancer have a 25%–30% likelihood of local recurrence and those with TNM stage III (Dukes' C) have a >50% probability of local recurrence. Local recurrence in patients with TNM stage I appears to be less than 10%.

Pre or postoperative radiation therapy significantly reduces the rate of local recurrence but does not appear to significantly affect long-term survival. Recent studies have demonstrated that postoperative combination radiation therapy and chemotherapy significantly improve patient survival and reduce both local and systemic postoperative recurrences in patients with TNM stage II (Dukes' B2) and TNM stage III (Dukes' C) rectal cancer.

## Current therapy for TNM stage II and III rectal cancer

Pre or postoperative radiation therapy combined with 5-fluorouracil (5-FU) and leucovorin, or 5-FU and levamisole. Adjuvant chemotherapy is usually well tolerated. This regimen is also used for metastatic disease, resulting in mild improvement in survival and quality of life.

## Side effects of 5-FU

### Common

Dermatitis, alopecia, stomatitis, nausea, vomiting, diarrhea, anorexia, and mucositis.

### Serious

Myelosuppression, hypotension, coronary ischemia, gastrointestinal ulceration, hepatitis, coagulopathy, and dyspnea.

## Side effects of levamisole

### Common

Nausea, vomiting, diarrhea, constipation, dermatitis, alopecia, fatigue, fever, arthralgia, and myalgia.

### Serious

Acute neurologic toxicity, myelosuppression, secondary infection, and depression.

## Side effects of leucovorin

Rare cases of allergic or anaphylactoid reactions have been reported.

## Side effects of radiation therapy

### Acute

Diarrhea, rectal pain, urgency, and urinary frequency.

### Chronic

Rectal bleeding, fecal incontinence, urgency, and diarrhea.

# Chapter 5.5

# Other rectal malignancies

## Carcinoid tumor

### Epidemiology

Carcinoid tumors are rare and occur in less than 0.001% of the general population. Only 12% originate in the rectum. The average age of presentation of rectal carcinoid tumors is 58 years, and they are equally common in men and women. Carcinoid tumors are seen in up to 10% of individuals with multiple endocrine neoplasia (MEN) syndrome.

### Pathophysiology

Carcinoid tumors arise from neuroendocrine cells of ectodermal origin. These cells are able to secrete a variety of hormones and other biologically active compounds. The tumors usually appear as small rectal nodules and are often found incidentally when small polyps are removed during routine colonoscopy.

### Symptoms

Carcinoid tumors are most often asymptomatic. However, symptoms such as rectal bleeding or rectal pain may be present. Advanced stage tumors may cause symptoms such as weight loss and anorexia.

### Diagnostic testing

Digital rectal examination may reveal a palpable nodule. Endoscopic evaluation and biopsy are required for diagnosis (see **Figure 1**).

### Treatment

Endoscopic-small lesions (<1 cm) may be removed in their entirety by endoscopy. Transanal resection may be performed for lesions <2 cm in diameter. Larger lesions are treated by rectal resection with anastomosis or abdominoperineal resection.

### Prognosis

Complete resection of lesions results in resolution of the disease. Lesions that are >2 cm in diameter have a high likelihood of metastasis (>60%), and patients may have carcinoid tumors in other portions of the bowel. Five-year survival is approximately 75% for all rectal carcinoid tumors.

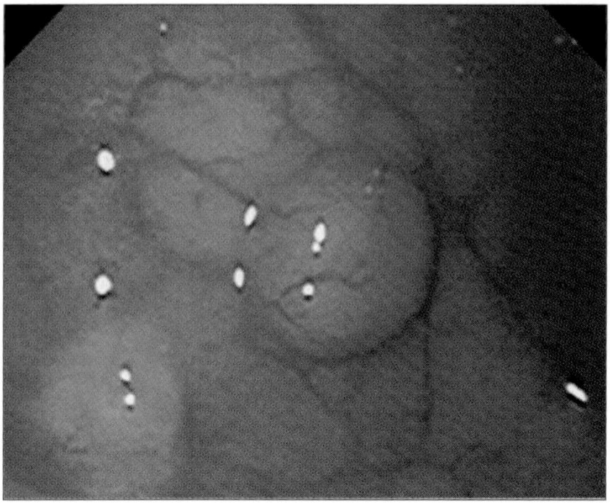

**Figure 1.** Polypoid colonic lesions without specific endoscopic appearances found to be a carcinoid tumor on histologic evaluation.

## Leiomyosarcoma

### Epidemiology
This is a rare colonic tumor that most often occurs in the rectum.

### Pathophysiology
Leiomyosarcoma is a slow-growing tumor that originates from intestinal smooth muscle cells. Local extension into perirectal tissue is a common finding.

### Symptoms
The most common symptoms are rectal pain and bleeding.

### Diagnosis
It is usually possible to detect the tumors on digital rectal examination. Endoscopy and biopsy are utilized to make the diagnosis.

### Treatment
Rectal resection is the treatment of choice.

### Prognosis
The predicted 5-year survival rate after diagnosis of leiomyosarcoma is 20%.

# Lymphoma

## Epidemiology

Primary rectal lymphoma is very rare (<0.1% of all malignant rectal neoplasms). Colonic lymphoma occurs most frequently in the cecum.

## Risk factors

Immunodeficiency syndromes, HIV infection, and, possibly, treatment with immunosuppressive agents.

## Treatment

Resection of the tumor alone or in combination with radiation therapy is used for primary intestinal lymphoma if there is no evidence of disease beyond the rectum. Otherwise, tumor staging followed by resection, chemotherapy and/or radiation therapy may be utilized.

# Metastatic rectal tumors

## Definition

Tumors that may metastasize or extend from the rectum. These tumors may metastasize locally to the prostate or uterus, or further a field to the ovaries, kidneys, pancreas, duodenum, stomach, breast, or lung.

## Symptoms

The main symptoms are rectal bleeding, rectal pain, and obstruction.

## Diagnosis

Digital rectal examination, endoscopy, and biopsy are utilized to make the diagnosis.

## Treatment

Usually palliative with fecal diversion if obstructive symptoms are present. Resection is reserved for intractable bleeding.

# Chapter 6

# Infectious disorders of the anus and rectum

# Chapter 6.1

# Chlamydia and lymphogranuloma venereum

## Organism

*Chlamydia trachomatis*. Twelve serologic variants (serovars) have been identified. Serovars D–K cause sexually transmitted urethritis and anorectal infections, and serovars L1–L3 cause lymphogranuloma venereum (LGV).

## Epidemiology

*C. trachomatis* infection is the most common sexually transmitted disease in the United States, and LGV is 20-times more common in men than in women.

## Patients at risk

Homosexual males, African–Americans, patients infected with HIV, and other people at risk of contracting venereal diseases, eg, people with multiple sex partners or people who are immunocompromised.

## Mode of transmission

Sexually transmitted.

## Incubation time

Clinical course. Several forms of *C. trachomatis* infection occur. Genital tract infection in males or females may be asymptomatic or result in the development of urethral discharge and/or dysuria, or ascending infections such as salpingitis. In males with LGV, a shallow ulcer first appears on the penis. Marked inguinal adenopathy (buboes) with fever, chills, and headache follow. Late stages of the disease are characterized by rectal or colorectal involvement (proctitis and colitis), rectal strictures, and rectovaginal fistulas. Proctocolitis may occur as the initial presentation in a severe form of the disease seen in homosexual males.

## Pathophysiology

Extensive inflammation results in diffuse infiltration, abscesses, and granuloma formation. Ulceration of the mucosa is seen on endoscopy.

## Diagnostic testing

Flexible sigmoidoscopy, biopsies, rectal culture, and microimmunofluorescent antibody or complement fixation testing.

## Treatment

The treatments for *C. trachomatis* infection are shown in **Table 1**.

| Treatment | Course |
|---|---|
| Azithromycin | Single dose of 1 g for 7 days |
| Doxycycline | 100 mg bid for 7 days |
| Tetracycline | 500 mg qid for 21 days |
| Erythromycin | 500 mg qid for 21 days |
| Trimethoprim-sulfamethoxazole | Double strength bid for 21 days |

**Table 1.** Treatments and their course for patients with *Chlamydia trachomatis* infection.

## Clinical pearls

Patients should be empirically treated for gonococcal proctitis if they are diagnosed with chlamydial proctitis. Sexual partners should also undergo treatment.

# Chapter 6.2

# Gonorrhea

## Organism

*Neisseria gonorrhoeae*, a Gram-negative, intracellular diplococcus.

## Epidemiology

From 400,000–800,000 cases of gonorrhea occur annually in the United States. There is an incidence of infection of 5% in high risk groups at any given time.

## Patients at risk

Homosexual males, particularly those practicing receptive anal intercourse; women with pelvic inflammatory disease; and males and females with other sexually transmitted diseases.

## Mode of transmission

Sexual intercourse, receptive anal intercourse, or spread from genital infection.

## Incubation time

Symptoms begin 5–7 days after exposure.

## Symptoms

### Typical

Diarrhea, mucopurulent discharge, and urgency.

### Additional

Arthritis, tenosynovitis, and skin rash.

## Pathophysiology

Infection causes inflammation of the rectum characterized by mucosal erosions, erythema, and friability.

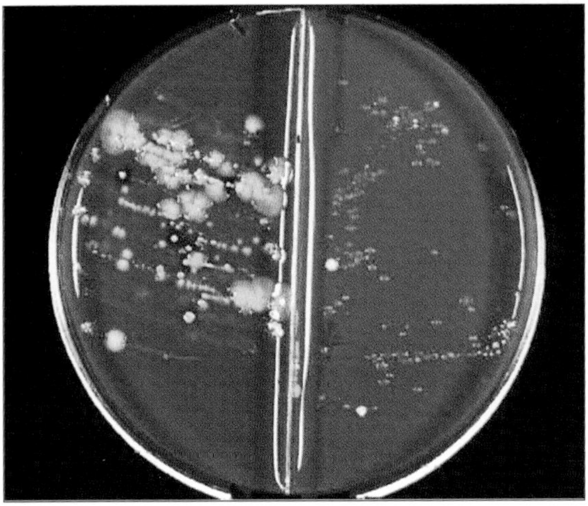

**Figure 1.** A Thayer-Martin biplate culture for *Neisseria gonorrhoeae*. The left side of the plate is chocolate agar; the right side contains chocolate agar plus antibiotics, which block growth of normal flora and allow the gonococcus to grow.

## Diagnostic tests

Rectal swab or biopsy testing with Gram-stain and culture using Thayer-Martin medium (see **Figure 1**).

## Treatment

The standard treatment is a single 250-mg dose of ceftriaxone administered intramuscularly. Patients should also receive treatment for possible concomitant chlamydial infection with, for example, 100 mg doxycycline bid for 21 days.

## Clinical pearls

Repeated cultures may be necessary due to difficulty in culturing *N. gonorrhoeae*. This condition is extremely common in homosexual males visiting sexually transmitted disease clinics.

# Chapter 6.3

# Herpes simplex

## Organism

Herpes simplex virus 2 (HSV-2).

## Epidemiology

Unlike human papilloma virus exposure, which commonly results in infection, perianal and rectal infection with herpes simplex is rare.

## Patients at risk

Homosexual males practicing receptive anal intercourse; people with multiple sex partners; and people with a prior history of genital herpes infection.

## Mode of transmission

Sexual or anal intercourse; may be spread from the mouth or gastrointestinal tract.

## Incubation time

From 2–7 days. It may be delayed by up to 3 weeks.

## Symptoms

Severe pain with defecation, tenesmus, diarrhea, mucopurulent discharge from rectum, and pruritus ani. Marked discomfort occurs with digital rectal examination or sigmoidoscopy.

## Pathophysiology

Initial symptoms may appear within a few days of exposure and include pruritus ani or paresthesia. Subsequently, vesicles form in the perianal region and rectum. Mucosal friability, ulcerations, and pustules may follow.

## Diagnostic testing

Sigmoidoscopy (usually performed with anesthesia because of discomfort) and/or scrapings or biopsies of anorectal ulcers for viral culture. Multinucleated giant cells with classic intranuclear inclusion bodies are seen on light microscopy.

## Treatment

The standard treatment is 400 mg oral acyclovir five times daily. Foscarnet is used for resistant cases.

## Clinical pearls

Biopsies or scrapings must be obtained from the edge of the ulcers, since organisms are not present in necrotic tissue and exudates in the central portion of the ulcers. Oral maintenance therapy with acyclovir is often used to suppress further herpes outbreaks.

# Chapter 6.4

# HIV-associated anorectal disease

## Epidemiology

Anorectal disorders have been described in 6%–33% of HIV-infected patients, and symptoms of anorectal disease are the most common indication (85%) for referral to surgery in this patient group. Approximately 50% of HIV-infected patients with anorectal disorders will require surgery.

## Patients at risk

High-risk groups for HIV infection include homosexual males and intravenous drug abusers. The incidence of sexually transmitted HIV has been increasing in the heterosexual population. Anorectal complications occur in the majority of HIV-infected homosexual males but are uncommon in HIV-positive intravenous drug abusers. Advanced HIV infection has been associated with the development of complex anal abscesses, chronic anal ulcers, and severe perianal sepsis. Anal malignancies associated with HIV occur almost exclusively in homosexual males.

## Symptoms

Symptoms vary according to individual conditions (see individual chapters for complete descriptions, including infectious conditions, neoplasms of the anus, anorectal abscess, perianal fistula, anal fissure, hemorrhoids, and diarrhea). Fecal incontinence in the absence of significant anorectal pathology may be seen in patients with late stage HIV infection as a result of severe diarrhea. Kaposi's sarcoma and non-Hodgkin's lymphoma generally present with pain, abscesses, or anorectal bleeding.

## Pathophysiology

Anorectal disorders in HIV-infected patients can be classified as:

1) Common anorectal pathology
2) Condylomata acuminata (venereal warts)
3) Perianal sepsis (including fistulas and abscesses)
4) Anorectal ulcerations
5) Anorectal malignancies (Kaposi's sarcoma, non-Hodgkin's lymphoma, and squamous cell carcinoma of the anal canal or anal margin)

Immunodeficiency often modifies the presentation of these diseases. For example, the development of anal abscesses in patients with advanced HIV infection may be associated with severe septic complications including necrotizing gangrene and "metastatic abscesses" in the liver, brain, and mediastinum. HIV infection is a definitive risk factor for the development of carcinoma *in situ* or invasive squamous cell carcinoma from anal or genital condylomata. Ulceration of the anal canal and perianal region is a unique manifestation of HIV infection.

## Diagnostic testing

Physical examination, flexible sigmoidoscopy with biopsy, and/or examination under anesthesia with biopsy.

## Treatment/clinical pearls

Treatments vary according to the condition. Anal abscesses are treated aggressively to prevent septic complications. Conservative management is suggested for anal fissures seen in patients with advanced HIV infection due to the risk of fecal incontinence and poor wound healing associated with surgical management. Hemorrhoids are also managed conservatively: rubber band ligation is to be avoided as cases of Fournier's gangrene (localized necrosis of the scrotum) have complicated this procedure in immunocompromised patients. This condition may develop when anaerobic organisms enter potential spaces in the groin following an initial infection at the banding site. Anal condylomata should be managed by surgical excision or fulguration instead of medical therapy due to the high-risk for the development of anorectal neoplasms in partially treated lesions.

Avoidance of receptive anal intercourse is suggested in patients with HIV-associated anal ulcerations. Intralesional steroids have been used for this condition. In general, conservative management of these conditions is recommended because of the risk of surgical complications and decreased wound healing in late-stage HIV infection.

# Chapter 6.5

# Syphilis

## Organism

*Treponema pallidum*.

## Epidemiology

The incidence of *T. pallidum* infection is increasing. Currently, 20 cases are seen per 100,000 people in the United States. The organism is highly contagious; 30%–50% of sexual partners of people infected with syphilis contract the disease.

## Patients at risk

Homosexual males practicing receptive anal intercourse and people with multiple sexual partners.

## Mode of transmission

Sexually transmitted.

## Incubation time

Two to eight weeks.

## Symptoms

May be relatively asymptomatic or produce severe anorectal discomfort, purulent anal discharge, difficulty with rectal evacuation, and tenesmus.

## Pathophysiology

The initial lesion is termed a "chancre" (primary syphilis), a well demarcated ulcer that begins at the site of infection. This progresses to disseminated anorectal disease characterized by ulceration, fissuring, fistulas, proctitis, and lymphadenopathy. A reddish rash due to systemic infection (secondary syphilis) follows after 2–10 weeks.

## Diagnostic testing

Anorectal swab with dark-field examination, serologic testing, and/or immunofluorescent staining.

## Treatment

Benzathine penicillin 2.4 million units intramuscularly, repeated after 7 days. Tetracycline (500 mg qid for 15 days) or erythromycin (500 mg qid for 30 days) are given to patients that are allergic to penicillin.

## Clinical pearls

Because this is a difficult infection to diagnose, patients with risk factors who are suspected of having anorectal syphilis should be treated empirically.

# Chapter 6.6

# Venereal warts (condylomata acuminata)

## Organism

Human papilloma DNA virus (HPV) from the papovavirus family. At least 60 subtypes of HPV have been identified. Of these subtypes, 6, 11, 16, 18, 31, 33, 35, 45, 51, 52, and 56 are sexually transmitted. Subtypes 16 and 18 are consistently associated with the development of cervical cancer.

## Epidemiology

HPV is the most common sexually transmitted viral infection. The incidence of condylomata acuminata is approximately 1 million per year in the United States. The condition is highly contagious; up to 70% of the sexual partners of those infected will contract the disease.

## Patients at risk

Sexual partners of infected individuals; sexually promiscuous people; homosexual males; patients with other sexually transmitted diseases such as gonorrhea, syphilis, and genital herpes; and victims of childhood sexual abuse.

## Mode of transmission

Sexual. All sexually transmitted subtypes are associated with the development of anogenital warts.

## Incubation time

Warts appear within 3–4 months of exposure to the virus.

## Symptoms

Fullness or a mass-like sensation in the perianal or genital region, pruritus ani, perianal or genital pain, rectal bleeding, and discharge.

## Pathophysiology

Anal infection causes squamous cell proliferation with multiple papillomas developing in the anal canal and urogenital area. Squamous metaplasia may occur with longstanding infection, particularly with HPV subtypes 16 and 18. After a number of years, carcinoma *in situ* with progression to invasive squamous cell carcinoma may develop with infections of subtypes 16 or 18.

## Diagnostic testing

Physical examination reveals characteristic findings: single or multiple warts with a cauliflower-like appearance are seen in the affected area (see **Figure 1**). The anal canal is affected in up to 90% of patients, and lesions frequently extend proximally to the dentate line. Biopsies show squamous cell proliferation and loss of the keratinized layer of the skin (acanthosis and hyperkeratosis). Proctoscopy or flexible sigmoidoscopy is required to determine the extent of anal and rectal involvement.

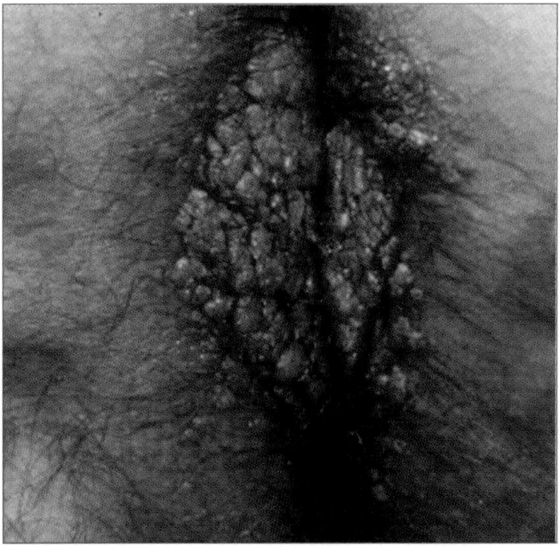

**Figure 1.** Physical examination shows cauliflower-like appearance of lesions.

## Treatment

### Topical therapy with destructive antiviral agents

Destruction of venereal warts with 25% podophyllin (a cytotoxic agent) in tincture of benzoin is a commonly performed, office-based procedure. After thorough cleansing, a small quantity is applied directly to the lesions (by a physician only). The solution is left in contact with the wart for 30 minutes during the first session, and for 1–4 hours during follow-up treatments, which are conducted weekly until either the warts are destroyed or the patient develops intolerance to treatment. The solution is removed from the area by cleansing with soap and water. The goal of the treatment is to completely destroy the warts. Physicians must be cautious when applying the tincture since application to large areas increases the risk of systemic absorption and toxicity.

Podofilox is an antimitotic agent, which is available in a 0.5% gel or topical solution. Podofilox can be applied to the affected area by the patient and is usually applied with a cotton tip. The patient should apply podofilox twice daily for 3 days and stop treatment for 4 days, resuming treatment on day 8. This weekly cycle is continued until complete elimination of warts has been achieved. In clinical trials, approximately 50% of patients achieved complete clearance of lesions after 2–4 weeks of treatment.

Imiquimod (Aldara) is an agent that promotes cytokine activity, thus increasing local antiviral immune activity. It is applied to the affected area three times per week and left in place for 6–10 hours. These treatments are continued until warts are cleared, or for up to 16 weeks. Treated areas may also be covered with nonocclusive dressings. Imiquimod has been demonstrated to be effective in more than 50% of patients using the medication.

### Other topical treatments

Cryotherapy, laser therapy, electrocoagulative therapy, injection of interferon and other cytotoxic agents into lesions.

### Surgical

Surgery is recommended for larger clusters of lesions, intrarectal lesions, refractory lesions, and recurrent lesions. Local anesthetic and epinephrine are injected into the base of the lesion(s) prior to removal with surgical scissors and forceps.

## Clinical pearls

Patients with smaller lesions and less extensive involvement are usually treated with the topical destructive agents podophyllin or podofilox. Patients who do not respond to these therapies (10%–50%) are referred for other forms of topical therapy or surgery. Some authors have suggested periodic surveillance for anal and genital cancer in affected individuals. Recurrence of symptoms should prompt immediate evaluation of the previously treated area. Recurrence of genital warts is a common phenomenon. Women with condylomata acuminata should undergo regular Pap smears since they are at high risk for the development of cervical dysplasia and carcinoma.

# Chapter 7

# Miscellaneous anorectal conditions

# Chapter 7.1

# Diarrhea

## Epidemiology

Self-limited diarrhea is extremely common. The passage of loose or watery stools without abdominal pain was found to occur in 4.3% of males and 2.2% of females surveyed in Bristol, UK during a 1-year period. Chronic diarrhea is thought to affect 5% of the adult population annually in the United States, and approximately 450,000 patients are hospitalized.

## Patients at risk

People with diabetes, celiac sprue, pancreatic disorders, or small intestinal disorders; travelers to Third World countries; HIV-infected patients; people on antibiotics; patients undergoing or having had radiation therapy; patients who have had surgery of the stomach, small intestine, or colon; and individuals receiving enteric formula feedings. A variety of medications and herbal preparations have laxative effects.

## Pathophysiology

Diarrhea occurs when the normal absorptive mechanism of the small intestine and colon is overwhelmed by excessive fluid secretion and hypermotility. The overall result is the passage of multiple frequent stools. Diarrhea is most objectively defined as the passage of more than 200 mL (200 g) of stool per day. Diarrhea can be divided into several categories, which are outlined below, together with common causes of each.

### Acute

Symptoms lasting from several days to 4 weeks. The majority of cases of acute diarrhea are due to viral, bacterial, or parasitic infection.

### Chronic

Symptoms lasting >4 weeks. A large number of conditions can result in the development of chronic diarrhea. Chronic diarrhea may be further divided into two main categories: osmotic diarrhea and secretory diarrhea.

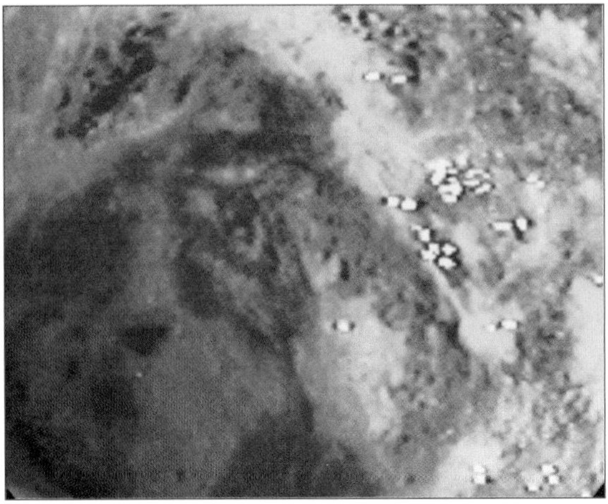

**Figure 1.** Infectious colitis due to cytomegalovirus in a patient with chronic myelogenous leukemia.

### Osmotic diarrhea

Malabsorbed or poorly absorbed sugars, other carbohydrates, and other osmotically active substances (such as magnesium) produce laxative effects by inducing the secretion of water. Since the overall osmolality of stool must remain at approximately 290 mosm/L, the presence of osmotically active substances in the colonic lumen results in net water secretion and increased stool volume.

### Secretory diarrhea

A variety of conditions – including hypermotility, infectious and inflammatory disorders, excessive secretion of chloride or bicarbonate, or decreased absorption of sodium – result in release of fluids and electrolytes.

## Symptoms

Passage of frequent watery or soft stools. Severe diarrhea may be associated with dehydration and consequent electrolyte disturbance. Frequent small stools with cramping and urgency suggest proctitis or left-sided colitis (see **Figure 1**). Large volume stools suggest a small intestinal source of diarrhea. Bloating, flatulence, and foul smelling and oily stools occur in malabsorptive states. Recent foreign travel suggests the presence of an infectious source.

## Diagnostic testing

A stool sample should be obtained, checked for parasites and *Clostridium difficile* toxin, and cultured. Other evaluations include fecal volume, fecal fat, electrolyte and pH measurement, complete blood count, serum chemistries, celiac sprue panel, thyroid stimulating hormone, flexible sigmoidoscopy, colonoscopy, small intestine biopsy, and 24-hour urine test for 5-HIAA (5-hydroxyindole acetic acid).

## Treatment

Identification of the underlying source of this symptom is critical for initiating proper therapy. It is best to control diarrhea by direct treatment of the cause. Treatments may include anti-inflammatory agents for inflammatory bowel disease and a gluten-free diet for celiac sprue. Treatments that may provide relief of the symptoms of diarrhea in the presence or absence of organic disorders include fiber, opioids, cholestyramine, octreotide, and anticholinergic agents.

## Clinical pearls

A careful history will assist in differentiating various causes of diarrhea. The possibility of laxative abuse should not be ignored. Patients with diarrhea and fecal incontinence generally experience improvement in their symptoms of incontinence when their diarrhea is under control.

# Chapter 7.2

# Fecal impaction

## Definition

Fecal impaction is the development of a colonic obstruction due to filling of the lumen with a large, hard stool. It occurs most commonly in the rectum.

## Epidemiology

The rising incidence of fecal impaction parallels the increasing prevalence of chronic constipation. Fecal impaction is the cause of colonic obstruction in up to 50% of bedridden patients in nursing homes and patients with spinal cord injuries.

## Patients at risk

Patients with spinal cord injuries and bedridden patients. Constipation may occur in up to 25% of the elderly population, and is three-times more common in women than in men. A variety of medications – including calcium channel blockers, anticholinergics, opioids, antidepressants, and antipsychotics – predispose to constipation and, therefore, the development of fecal impaction. A number of neurologic diseases (Parkinson's disease, dementia, multiple sclerosis) are associated with decreased colonic function and constipation, therefore placing patients at risk for fecal impaction. Endocrine disorders including diabetes and hypothyroidism are additional risk factors. Dehydration increases the likelihood of developing fecal impaction in high-risk patients.

## Symptoms

Constipation, rectal pain, and a sensation of a rectal mass are common symptoms. Other symptoms, including diarrhea and fecal incontinence due to overflow of liquid stool past the impacted fecal bolus, may be present. Patients with neurologic diseases or spinal cord injury may be unaware of the presence of the fecal impaction. In addition, fecal impaction in patients with spinal cord injury may lead to autonomic dysreflexia, a medical emergency characterized by the acute development of symptomatic hypertension with hyperactive reflexes. Rectal bleeding may occur in patients with stercoral ulcers (see **Pathophysiology**). In extreme cases of fecal impaction, colonic obstruction with abdominal distention and signs and symptoms of bowel perforation or peritonitis may be present.

## Pathophysiology

Decreased neuromuscular function of the colon results in colonic hypomotility, prolonged transit time in the colon, and fecal retention. Increased contact time between fecal material and the colon results in firm, dehydrated stools. A vicious cycle may develop in which increasing stool retention further delays motility and produces even drier, firmer stools. Altered sensorium may exacerbate the problem through the loss of normal impulses to defecate. A hard stool may be retained for such a prolonged period of time in a single segment of the colon that ischemic ulceration – a stercoral ulcer – may occur.

## Diagnostic testing

Examination of the abdomen may reveal the presence of soft or firm masses, particularly over the left colon. Digital rectal examination will reveal a firm, mobile mass in the rectum. An abdominal x-ray will demonstrate the presence of stool accumulation in the colon. A sigmoidoscopy may be required to rule out other types of rectal mass, eg, carcinoma.

## Treatment

Most forms of fecal impaction can be treated with digital fecal disimpaction. However, this procedure may produce marked discomfort and even hypotension in some patients, and, therefore, some form of sedation should be considered. Following the removal of the largest and most obstructive fecal boluses, follow-up with gentle enema therapy is performed. In patients who have developed fecal impaction, a bowel regimen including laxatives and enemas on a regular basis is suggested.

## Clinical pearls

It is particularly important to remind patients who are on medications that cause constipation to consume large volumes of liquid on a daily basis, for example 5–8 glasses of water or other nonalcoholic fluids daily. Patients who have an episode of fecal impaction should be placed on a regular regimen of stool softeners and/or osmotic laxatives as a prophylaxis against further episodes.

# Chapter 7.3

# Ileoanal pouch anastomosis

## General description

In patients requiring proctocolectomy, ileoanal pouch anastomosis has obviated the need for ileostomy as it preserves fecal continence. A direct anastomosis between the ileum and anus was first performed in 1968. In 1978, creation of an "S pouch", which functions as a reservoir, was incorporated into the procedure. The J pouch, which is currently the most commonly performed procedure, was introduced in 1980. Ileoanal pouch anastomosis after creation of a J or S pouch is now the procedure of choice in appropriate patients requiring complete removal of the colon (see **Figure 1**).

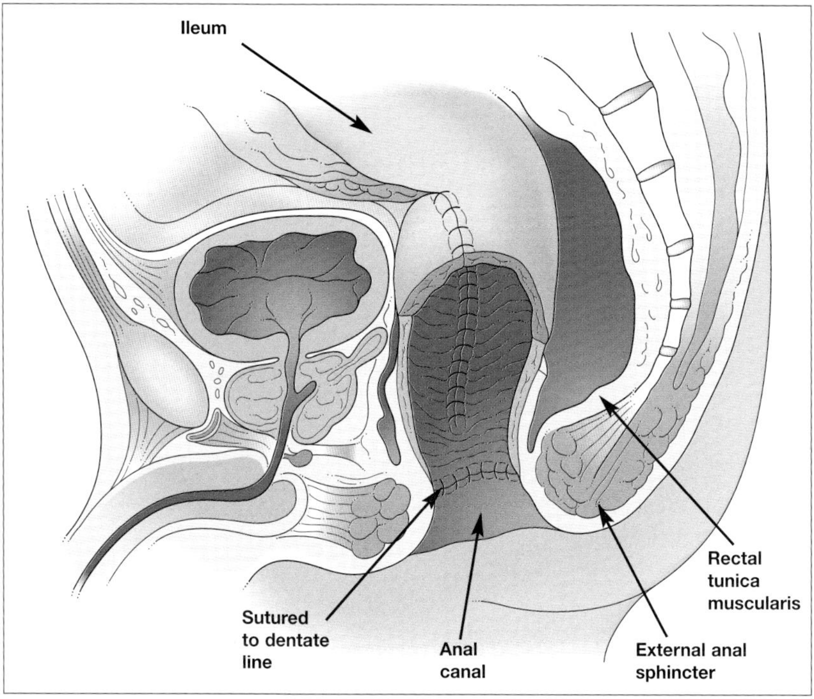


**Figure 1.** Diagram of ileoanal pouch anastomosis.

The indications, relative contraindications, and contraindications to this procedure are outlined in **Table 1**.

| Indications | Contraindications | Relative contraindications |
|---|---|---|
| Chronic ulcerative colitis | Crohn's disease | Massive obesity |
| Familial adenomatous polyposis | Cancer of the distal rectum | Emergency operation |
| Multiple colorectal malignancies | Poor anal sphincter function | Use of steroid medication |
| | Anal sphincter excised | Indeterminate colitis |
| | Age >65 years | |

**Table 1.** Indications and contraindications for ileoanal pouch anastomosis.

## Alternative procedures

End ileostomy (Brook ileostomy) or continent ileostomy (Kock pouch).

## How the procedure is performed

This procedure may be carried out in one, two, or three stages depending on the preference of the performing surgeon and the general condition of the patient. For example, in a patient with severe acute colitis, a colectomy and loop ileostomy may be created for the first stage. After 3–6 months, when the patient is physically and nutritionally improved, a proctectomy is performed with creation of a J pouch. Finally, in the third stage of the procedure, the loop ileostomy is closed.

The first stage in the procedure is a total abdominal colectomy (some centers perform the colectomy laparoscopically). The rectum is then dissected within the pelvis through the dilated anal canal; the surgeon must be especially cautious during this stage of the procedure to preserve the anal sphincter, local portions of the genitourinary systems, and perineal nerves. The distal 15 cm of the ileum is divided and then folded back onto itself (in a J shape) and opened to produce a reservoir. Temporary ileostomy may be performed to protect the pouch and then closed on a later occasion. The ileoanal anastomosis may be hand sewn or stapled; a double-stapled technique is utilized for stapled anastomosis (see **Figure 2**).

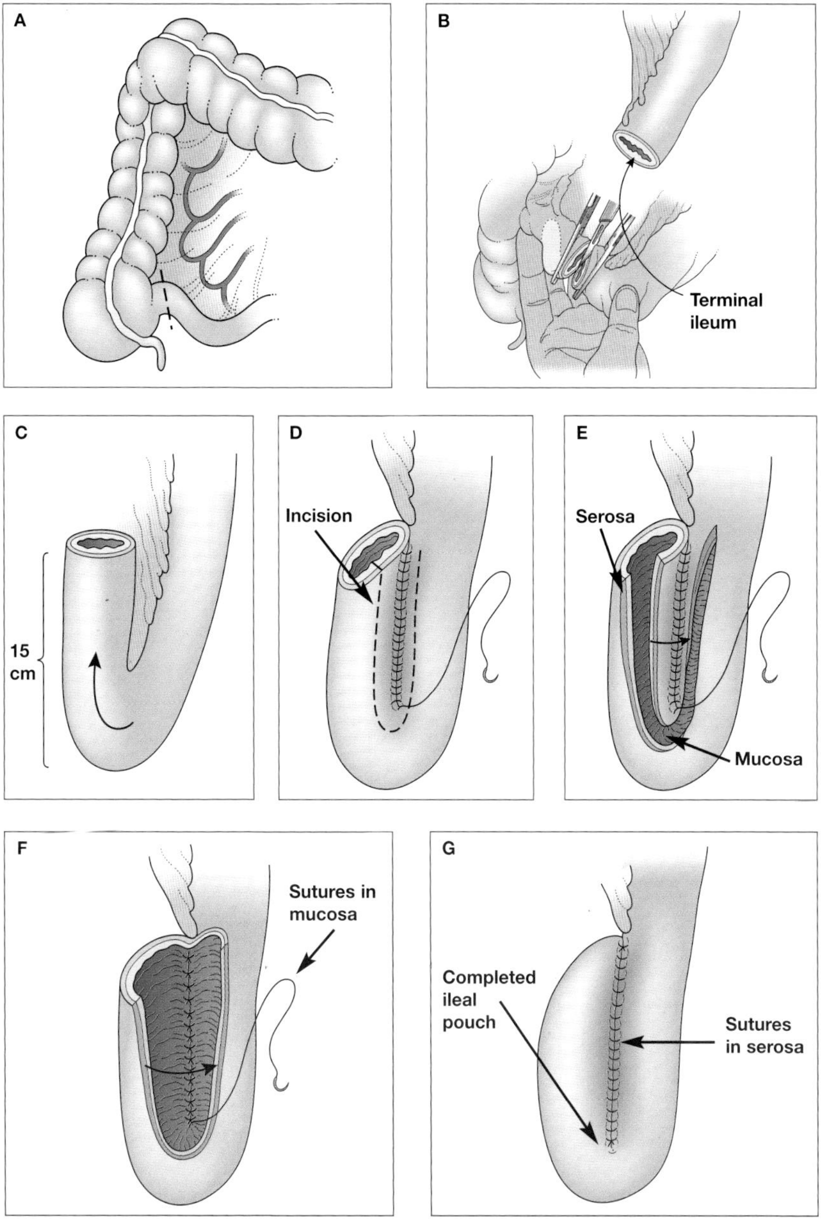


**Figure 2.** Construction of J-shaped ileal pouch. **(A, B)** The terminal ileum is divided and the colon is removed. **(C)** The terminal ileum is fashioned into a J-shape with 15-cm limbs. **(D, E)** The antimesenteric border of ileum is divided. **(F)** The posterior mucosal layer of pouch is sutured. **(G)** The pouch is completed.

## Results obtained

More than 90% of patients report satisfaction with their procedure. Mild fecal incontinence, particularly with spotting of stool in the underclothing at night, occurs chronically in up to 50% of patients having this procedure, and approximately 25% of patients with an ileoanal pouch anastomosis will wear a pad to prevent soiling of underclothing.

## Complications

### Surgical

Approximately 30% of patients who undergo this ileoanal pouch anastomosis will experience a surgical complication. Anastomotic leakage occurs in about 10% of patients undergoing this procedure (see **Figure 3**). This is managed with intravenous antibiotics, drainage of pelvic fluid, and bowel rest. Abdominal sepsis, which occurs in <5% of patients who have an ileoanal pouch anastomosis, often results in pouch failure and excision. These patients then require a permanent ileostomy. Small bowel obstruction is seen in approximately 20% of patients and requires additional surgery in about half of these. Anastomotic strictures are common (5%–15% of patients) and are usually easily managed with digital dilatation or insertion of Hegar's dilators. Surgical repair of strictures with revision of the ileoanal anastomosis is necessary in a small number of cases.

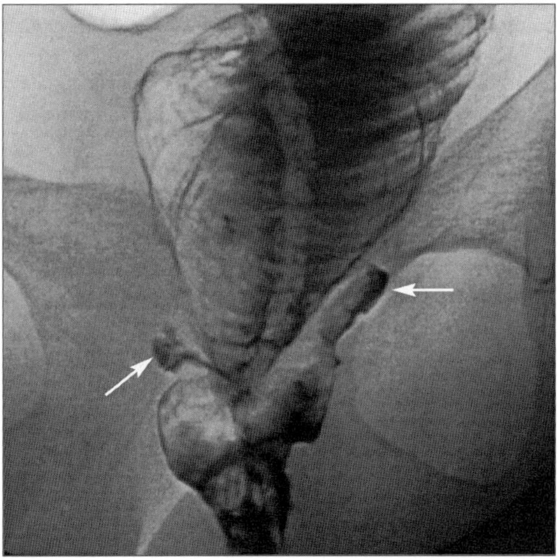

**Figure 3.** Ileoanal pouch anastomosis. Several small anastomotic leaks are demonstrated on dynamic proctography (arrows).

## Long-term

Fecal leakage and incontinence as described in the **Results obtained** section above. The other long-term complication of ileoanal pouch anastomosis is sexual dysfunction. Male patients report a 2% prevalence of impotence and a 2%–4% prevalence of retrograde ejaculation. Although a small percentage of women complain of dyspareunia (difficult or painful coitus), 50% report improved sexual function following the procedure.

### *Pouchitis*

This is a nonspecific inflammatory disorder. Symptoms include watery diarrhea, passage of blood, and cramping of the abdomen. In some patients, pouchitis is associated with systemic symptoms such as fever and arthralgia.

Mucosal edema, granularity, and/or ulcerations may be seen endoscopically in the affected pouch. The etiology of pouchitis has not been fully determined. The condition may represent overgrowth of anaerobic bacteria within the pouch, decreased mucosal exposure to intraluminal nutrients, or autoimmune induced inflammation. Pouchitis occurs in 20%–50% of patients who receive ileoanal pouch anastomosis for ulcerative colitis, but rarely in patients who undergo the procedure due to familial polyposis coli. Episodes occur most commonly within the first 6 months following creation of the pouch. In 39% of patients, only a single acute episode occurs.

Five percent of patients develop recurrent or chronic pouchitis. About half of these patients will need resection of the pouch. The standard treatment is metronidazole (10–20 mg/kg/day), sometimes in combination with ciprofloxacin (500 mg, bid). Treatment duration is usually 2–4 weeks. Chronic pouchitis has been treated with 5-ASA (5-acetylsalicylic acid) containing agents such as Pentasa or mesalamine enemas, and immunosuppressant drugs, eg, corticosteroids azathioprine, short-chain fatty acid enemas, and probiotics. Administration of live probiotic bacteria has been demonstrated to maintain remission in patients with chronic pouchitis.

### *Dysplasia and cancer*

Depending on the type of rectal dissection performed, a small portion of the rectal mucosa from the anal transition zone can be left at the site of the anastomosis. This cuff of rectal tissue is larger when a double-stapled technique is used. Although rare, dysplasia and carcinoma have been reported in this remaining portion of rectum mucosa. Current recommendations include surveillance sigmoidoscopy with biopsies at the site of the anastomosis every 1–3 years.

## Clinical pearls

Patients with symptoms of pouchitis require a careful history and endoscopic evaluation with biopsies to confirm the diagnosis. Other entities that mimic symptoms of pouchitis include acute gastroenteritis and recurrent inflammatory bowel disease (Crohn's disease). Adaptation with improvement of pouch function, as demonstrated by decreased stool frequency and increased fluid and electrolyte absorption, occurs during the first 6–12 months following pouch construction.

# Chapter 7.4

# Pilonidal sinuses

## Epidemiology

Symptomatic pilonidal sinuses generally develop between the ages of 20 and 30 years. Three-quarters of cases are seen in males. There is some suggestion that trauma to the skin overlying the sacrococcygeal region (such as strenuous activity and sitting in vehicles in rugged environments – as seen in military personnel) may increase the likelihood of development of the condition.

## Symptoms

If an abscess is present, pain may be the predominant symptom. Otherwise, patients will notice swelling, drainage, and tenderness of the affected area.

## Pathophysiology

Pilonidal sinuses develop in the intergluteal cleft and in the skin overlying the sacrum and coccygeal bone (see **Figure 1**). The condition develops when a sinus tract forms following an episode of folliculitis and abscess formation. The initiating factor may be a plug of keratin that develops in the hair follicle. Shafts of hair entering a previously developed sinus may also initiate the condition. Recurrent abscesses, infection, and multiple sinus tracts may be seen.

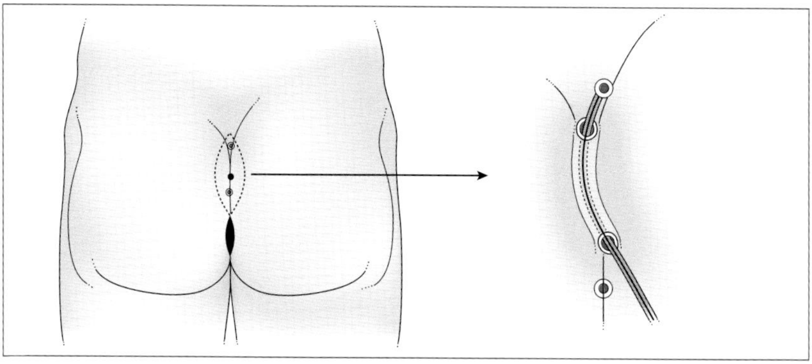

**Figure 1.** Pilonidal sinuses. On examination, pits or external openings in the intergluteal cleft are seen. The openings often communicate with each other, as shown on the right.

## Diagnosis

Physical examination reveals an area of inflammation, tenderness, and erythema in the gluteal crease, usually 5–7 cm from the anal opening. Hair follicles will often be noted at the site of the lesion and there is often more than one sinus opening. The presence of hair follicles and the lack of an opening from within the anorectal region differentiate pilonidal cysts from anal and rectal fistulas.

## Treatment

If an abscess is present, incision and drainage are the treatments of choice, followed by complete excision when the acute process is resolved. Shaving hair from the intergluteal cleft on a weekly basis decreases the chance of recurrence.

## Clinical pearls

Recurrences following excision of the pilonidal sinus need additional excisions. In refractory cases, more extensive excision surgery may be required.

# Chapter 7.5

# Rectal foreign bodies

## Epidemiology

The majority of the foreign bodies found in the rectum have been placed there rectally; however, swallowed objects may occasionally lodge in the rectum. Foreign bodies may be introduced either intentionally (autoeroticism, sexual activity, rape) or unintentionally (as a means of dislodging impacted stool).

## Patients at risk

Homosexuals; individuals practicing receptive anal sex utilizing foreign objects; rape victims; children; people with altered sensorium; and patients with rectal or anal strictures (in the case of swallowed objects).

## Pathophysiology

After placing large objects in the rectum, intense anal spasm and/or pain sometimes prevent simple removal.

A sharp swallowed object may lodge itself in normal rectal mucosa. Other swallowed objects may become impacted at the rectosigmoid junction. Narrowed luminal caliber secondary to strictures or diverticular disease increases the likelihood of impaction.

## Symptoms

Pain in the abdomen or rectum, rectal bleeding, discharge, and symptoms of peritonitis (abdominal distention, fever, peritoneal signs).

## Diagnostic testing

Physical examination should include careful abdominal examination to rule out peritonitis. The abdomen should be palpated for masses and the anus should be carefully inspected for evidence of fissure and/or anal trauma. Prior to the performance of a rectal examination, an abdominal x-ray should be performed (see **Figure 1**). Subsequently a digital rectal exam can be carefully performed (as long as a sharp object is not suspected). Assessment of anal sphincter tone is recommended. Patients may require anesthesia for adequate examination.

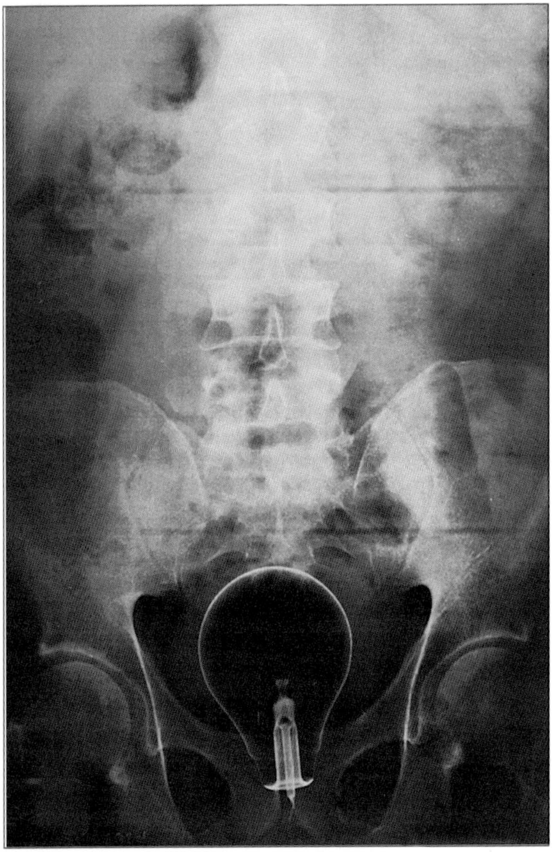

**Figure 1.** Rectal foreign body (light bulb) demonstrated on abdominal radiograph.

## Treatment

Following adequate anesthesia, small objects may be digitally removed. Endoscopic removal may be possible in selected cases; removal of sharp objects requires an overtube. General anesthesia is used for the removal of larger objects. This can be performed using a variety of devices including obstetric forceps and modified padded pliers. After the insertion of a rigid proctoscope, a Foley catheter or a Sengstaken–Blakemore tube may be inflated proximal to the object, which is then pulled down towards the anus. Patients who have evidence of peritonitis will require laparotomy.

## Clinical pearls

The rectosigmoid region should be visualized endoscopically following removal of a foreign object to ensure that it has been completely removed and to rule out mucosal injury.

# Chapter 8

# Patient information

# Chapter 8.1

# Anal fissure

## What is an anal fissure?

An anal fissure is a tear or crack in the lining of the anal canal.

## How does an anal fissure develop?

Anal fissures are believed to start with passage of a large, hard bowel movement that results in tearing of the skin (anoderm) of the anal canal. Excess contraction or spasm of the anal sphincter and weakening of the area where the fissure develops can contribute to the condition. In time, if the fissure does not heal, a chronic anal fissure or ulcer may develop.

## What are the symptoms of an anal fissure?

The most common symptoms of an anal fissure are pain during the process of defecation and after completion of the bowel movement. Minor bleeding from the anus may occur. With time, pain and pressure in the anal area may become more continuous and severe.

## Are there any other conditions that cause the same symptoms as an anal fissure?

Thrombosed hemorrhoids may mimic the symptoms of an anal fissure. Other diseases of the anus, such as infections and tumors, may have similar symptoms.

## What factors increase the risk of developing an anal fissure?

Anal fissures may occur in association with Crohn's disease, anal and rectal infections, AIDS, and tumors of the anus. Constipation, straining, and passage of hard bowel movements may initiate the development of an anal fissure. A low fiber, high fat diet may predispose to the condition.

## Can anal fissures predispose to cancer?

No.

## What tests are performed to diagnose anal fissures?

A physical examination of the anus is often enough to make the diagnosis. Sometimes, an anoscope or sigmoidoscope may be used to assist with the diagnosis.

### What over-the-counter treatments or home remedies can be used for anal fissures?

Stool softeners such as dioctyl sodium sulfosuccinate (Colace); bulking agents such as psyllium (Metamucil, Konsyl), methylcellulose (Citrucel), or calcium polycarbophyl (FiberCon, Konsyl); local anesthetic creams containing lidocaine (Analpram, Lidomantle, Tronolane).

### What prescription medications are used for anal fissures and how do they work?

Nitroglycerin ointment may relax the anal sphincter and allow the fissure to heal.

### What nonsurgical procedures can be used to treat anal fissures?

Botulinum toxin (Botox) injections into the anal sphincter may be used. These cause relaxation of the sphincter and allow for better healing of the fissure. Anal dilatation (stretching of the anal muscle) using a finger or dilating device is sometimes used.

### Is surgery ever used as a treatment for anal fissures?

Yes.

### When is surgery used to treat anal fissures?

When symptoms persist despite medical therapy and/or Botox injections.

### What surgical procedures are performed for the treatment of anal fissure?

Lateral sphincterotomy (making a small incision into the internal anal sphincter). This may be accompanied by surgical removal of the fissure itself.

### What additional information should I know about anal fissures?

Anal fissures may occur at any age and are even seen in infants. New medical therapies (nitroglycerin ointment, Botox) have helped many patients avoid the need for surgery for this condition.

# Chapter 8.2

# Fecal incontinence

### What is fecal incontinence?

Fecal incontinence involves the loss of rectal contents including gas, mucus, or stool without awareness or control of the occurrence.

### How does fecal incontinence occur?

As a result of damage to the nerves and muscles that normally control the function of the anus and rectum. Fecal incontinence may also be present in persons with brain or spinal cord damage. Severe or frequent diarrhea may overwhelm the anal sphincter and cause leakage.

### What are the symptoms of fecal incontinence?

Inability to control passage of stool or gas. Fecal incontinence is often characterized by soiling of clothing and bedding.

### Are there any other conditions that cause the same symptoms as fecal incontinence?

Colitis, proctitis, and anal or rectal infection.

### What factors increase the risk of developing fecal incontinence?

Aging, prior surgery of the anus, trauma to the anus, injury to the anal muscles during delivery of a baby, neurologic diseases, brain damage, mental retardation.

### Can fecal incontinence predispose to cancer?

No.

### What tests are performed to diagnose fecal incontinence?

Anorectal manometry, anorectal ultrasound, anorectal electromyography (EMG), defecography.

### What over-the-counter treatments or home remedies can be used for fecal incontinence?

Fiber supplements, especially calcium polycarbophyl tablets (FiberCon, Konsyl), or loperamide (Imodium). The elimination of dairy products from the diet may improve symptoms.

### What prescription medications are used for fecal incontinence and how do they work?

Hyoscyamine (Levbid, NuLev), dicyclomine (Bentyl), clindium, and atropine (Lomotil); opiates such as codeine, cholestyramine (Questran). These drugs produce constipation by slowing the movement of the intestine and promoting increased fluid absorption. When the stools are dry and firm, they are less likely to leak out of the anus.

### What nonsurgical procedures can be used to treat fecal incontinence?

Biofeedback therapy, a form of relaxation therapy and training of the anal sphincter, may be effective in improving the symptoms. A new outpatient technique called Secca has been introduced in the United States. The Secca procedure delivers radiofrequency waves into the anal sphincter to remodel and tighten the muscle.

### Is surgery ever used as a treatment for fecal incontinence?

Yes.

### When is surgery used to treat fecal incontinence?

When symptoms cannot be controlled with the above named therapies. Surgery is generally reserved for a small number of patients with the condition. For example, the best results with surgery are seen in patients with a deformity of the sphincter due to damage from childbirth or previous surgery. All other operations for fecal incontinence should be considered new or experimental and are usually performed at specialized surgical centers.

### What surgical procedures are performed for the treatment of fecal incontinence?

Repair of the damaged sphincter muscle, transplantation of another muscle to replace the damaged anus, colostomy to divert the stool into a bag to prevent leakage from the anus.

### What additional information should I know about fecal incontinence?

This condition occurs in up to 1% of individuals who are over 65 years old.

# Chapter 8.3

# Hemorrhoids

*(also known as: piles)*

### What are hemorrhoids?

Hemorrhoids are enlarged veins around the anus. They may be located either inside the rectum (internal hemorrhoids), or within or outside of the anal canal (external hemorrhoids).

### How do hemorrhoids occur?

Straining on the toilet and aging cause enlargement of the veins and loosening of their supporting structure.

### What are the symptoms of hemorrhoids?

Internal hemorrhoids cause bleeding, pressure around the anus, soiling, and, occasionally, severe pain.

External hemorrhoids primarily cause pain, itching, and discomfort.

### Are there any other conditions that cause the same symptoms as hemorrhoids?

Anal fissure, anal fistula, venereal warts, and tumors of the rectum and anal canal can mimic the symptoms of hemorrhoids. It is particularly important to notify your physician should you develop rectal bleeding. This symptom should not be dismissed as being caused by hemorrhoids without a full evaluation.

### What factors increase the risk of developing hemorrhoids?

Constipation, straining, and childbirth.

### Can hemorrhoids predispose to developing cancer?

No.

### What tests are performed to diagnose hemorrhoids?

Physical examination, anoscopy, and flexible sigmoidoscopy.

### What over-the-counter treatments or home remedies can be used for hemorrhoids?

Dietary fiber; fiber supplements such as psyllium husk (Metamucil, Konsyl), methylcellulose (Citrucel), calcium polycarbophyl (FiberCon, Konsyl); sitz baths; local anesthetic creams (Anusol, Preparation H, ProctoCream); stool softeners.

### What prescription medications are used for hemorrhoids and how do they work?

Local anesthetic creams and ointments containing hydrocortisone (ProctoCream, Anusol, Lidomantle). These medications reduce swelling of the dilated veins and decrease inflammation around the hemorrhoids.

### What nonsurgical procedures can be used to treat hemorrhoids?

For internal hemorrhoids only: rubber band ligation, injection with a sclerosing agent or saline, photocoagulation, cryosurgery, or electrical coagulation.

### Is surgery ever used as a treatment for hemorrhoids?

Yes.

### When is surgery used to treat hemorrhoids?

Internal hemorrhoids: when the hemorrhoids protrude out of the anus to a marked degree, even without straining.

External hemorrhoids: a clot may be surgically removed if it causes severe pain (the clot should be removed within 48 hours of onset of pain. After 48 hours, the entire hemorrhoid should be removed in order to relieve severe pain).

### What surgical procedures are performed for the treatment of hemorrhoids?

Removal of the hemorrhoidal bundle. Sometimes this is accompanied by stretching of the anus and/or cutting the internal sphincter muscle.

### What additional information should I know about hemorrhoids?

Hemorrhoids occur in up to 50% of the adult population. Treatment with the recommended over-the-counter remedies is effective for most patients with hemorrhoids.

# Chapter 8.4

# Kegel exercises

## What are Kegel exercises?

Kegel exercises are a form of pelvic muscle strengthening technique that have been developed to assist with the treatment of fecal and urinary incontinence.

## What is the purpose of performing Kegel exercises?

Many individuals with fecal or urinary incontinence have weak pelvic muscles. This results in less tensile strength for withholding stool and urine. In addition, the pelvic muscles form a strong basket-like sling, which secures the bladder, vagina, and rectum in place within the pelvis. When these muscles weaken, the function of these organs may diminish. This can lead to further muscle weakening and nerve damage of the area. Strengthening the pelvic muscles will limit the progression of this problem and has been shown to improve the symptoms of fecal and urinary incontinence.

## What causes weakening of the pelvic muscles?

The normal aging process leads to decreased pelvic muscle tone. Affected muscles include the anal sphincter and the muscles of the pelvic wall. Other factors that can result in weakening of the pelvic muscles include obesity, childbirth, lifting of heavy objects, diabetes, rheumatoid disorders, and neurologic disorders such as Parkinson's disease and multiple sclerosis.

## How are Kegel exercises performed?

These can be performed in several ways:

1) Lie on your back with your knees bent and pulled in towards your chest. "Hug" your knees so that the left hand is holding the right knee and the right hand is holding the left knee. Contract your abdomen and squeeze the buttocks together and hold for 10–20 seconds. Repeat this technique two or three times per day.
2) While urinating, use your muscles to start and stop urination. Perform this same muscle squeezing technique while not urinating: hold the squeeze for 5–10 seconds and relax. Repeat this 10–20 times. Perform this technique three or four times per day.

3) While sitting in a relaxed position with the legs bent, take a deep breath and squeeze the buttocks together and tighten the anus. Hold this position for 5–10 seconds. Relax and repeat three to four times. Perform this exercise three or four times per day.
4) While in a standing position, squeeze the buttocks and contract and hold in your abdomen. Hold in place for 10 seconds. Repeat this three to five times. Perform this exercise three or four times per day.
5) Special cones have been developed as an aid for tightening the vaginal muscles. They come in various sizes and are held in place by squeezing the vagina. The cones should be held for about 15 minutes and this exercise should be repeated two to four times per day.

Any or all of the above techniques can be used to strengthen the pelvic muscles. It is important to choose an exercise regimen that you are comfortable with and can be easily performed on a regular basis.

### How soon will I notice a benefit from performing Kegel exercises?

Some improvement may be noticed within several weeks. However, it may take 3–6 months to have full benefit from these exercises.

### What additional information should I know about Kegel exercises?

These exercises may make childbirth easier when performed during pregnancy in preparation for labor. Some women have reported that regular performance of Kegel exercises results in improved sexual function and responsiveness.

# Chapter 8.5

# Nonrelaxing puborectalis syndrome

*(also known as: anismus and paradoxical puborectalis contraction)*

## What is nonrelaxing puborectalis syndrome?

Nonrelaxing puborectalis syndrome is a benign condition that causes chronic constipation.

## How does nonrelaxing puborectalis syndrome occur?

In this condition, one of the anorectal muscles – the puborectalis, which is important for defecation – is not functioning properly. The puborectalis muscle keeps the stool from exiting the rectum until the proper time for defecation. This muscle is normally contracted. At the time of defecation, the puborectalis muscle relaxes, allowing stool to pass from the rectum. In patients with nonrelaxing puborectalis syndrome, this muscle is unable to relax at the time of defecation, therefore, the stool remains locked within the rectum.

## What are the symptoms of nonrelaxing puborectalis syndrome?

Constipation, straining, and difficulty with evacuation.

## Are there any other conditions that cause the same symptoms as nonrelaxing puborectalis syndrome?

Mechanical obstruction or blockage of the anorectal region can cause similar symptoms. Causes of blockage include anal strictures (benign), Crohn's disease, and cancers. Other causes of constipation that have similar symptoms include rectoceles and other pelvic floor disorders.

## What factors increase the risk of developing nonrelaxing puborectalis syndrome?

Anxiety and excessive attention to bowel habits may be causative factors in some patients with this condition. However, the link between these factors and the onset of nonrelaxing puborectalis syndrome is not fully understood.

## Can nonrelaxing puborectalis syndrome predispose to cancer?

No.

### What tests are performed to diagnose nonrelaxing puborectalis syndrome?

A physical examination is sometimes enough to make this diagnosis. However, most physicians will suggest other tests which may include anorectal manometry, defecography, and anorectal electromyography.

### What over-the-counter treatments or home remedies can be used for nonrelaxing puborectalis syndrome?

A high fiber diet, or high-dose fiber supplements such as psyllium (Metamucil, Konsyl) and methylcellulose (Citrucel), is helpful in a small number of patients. Milk of magnesia and stool softeners are beneficial in some patients.

### What prescription medications are used for nonrelaxing puborectalis syndrome and how do they work?

Laxatives such as polyethylene glycol (MiraLax) and lactulose may be beneficial.

### What nonsurgical procedures can be used to treat nonrelaxing puborectalis syndrome?

Biofeedback therapy has been shown to be effective in up to 90% of patients with nonrelaxing puborectalis syndrome. This therapy consists of relaxation techniques and exercises that are taught in conjunction with measurement of the contraction and relaxation of the anorectal muscles. Botulinum toxin (Botox) injections into the anal sphincter or puborectalis muscle have been shown to be beneficial in the small group of patients that have been given this treatment thus far.

### Is surgery ever used as a treatment for nonrelaxing puborectalis syndrome?

A very small number of patients have apparently benefited from surgery for this condition. However, no surgery has been proven to be effective for the majority of patients with nonrelaxing puborectalis syndrome.

### When is surgery used to treat nonrelaxing puborectalis syndrome?

When dietary changes, fiber supplementation, laxatives, biofeedback therapy, and Botox treatments have failed.

### What surgical procedures are performed for the treatment of nonrelaxing puborectalis syndrome?

Dilatation or stretching of the anus with special catheters has been tried and has been successful in a study of a small group of patients. Another surgical technique used occasionally for this condition involves cutting the puborectalis muscle to decrease its function.

### What additional information should I know about nonrelaxing puborectalis syndrome?

Some patients with this condition may be incorrectly diagnosed with irritable bowel syndrome. Although patients may be skeptical regarding the benefits of biofeedback therapy, at present it appears to be the best treatment for nonrelaxing puborectalis syndrome.

# Chapter 8.6

# Perianal Crohn's disease

## What is perianal Crohn's disease?

Perianal Crohn's disease refers to the occurrence of thickened skin tags, fissures, fistulas, and abscesses in the anus and skin that surrounds the anal region.

## How does perianal Crohn's disease occur?

When Crohn's disease affects the glands of the anus, the inflammation and tissue damage can spread to the skin and nearby structures. Infections may occur in the inflamed areas causing abscesses. Healing of the inflamed areas may leave fibrous tracks connecting the anus or rectum to the skin. Narrowing of the anal opening can occur due to scar formation.

## What are the symptoms of perianal Crohn's disease?

Although perianal involvement can occur in up to 35% of people with Crohn's disease, it is often asymptomatic. When present, symptoms include anal itching (pruritus ani) and mild discomfort around the anus. Swelling, due to enlarged anal skin tags, may be noticed by some patients. Abscesses may cause pain and fever. Sinus tracks (which connect internal inflamed and infected areas to the skin) may drain from the perianal region.

## Are there any other conditions that cause the same symptoms as perianal Crohn's disease?

Anal fissures and fistulas may occur in patients without Crohn's disease. Infections of the perianal region and rectum may have similar symptoms. Occasionally, anal cancer can present with swelling and/or fistulization in the anal region.

## What factors increase the risk of developing perianal Crohn's disease?

Crohn's disease of the lower intestine is the most common precursor to perianal Crohn's disease. More rarely, it is seen in patients with Crohn's disease of the small intestine.

## Can perianal Crohn's disease predispose to cancer?

Yes, but very rarely. If you have perianal Crohn's disease and develop bleeding or marked worsening of your symptoms, you should report this to your physician.

### What tests are performed to diagnose perianal Crohn's disease?

A physical examination is often sufficient to make this diagnosis. If the disease appears to be complicated, a magnetic resonance image (MRI) of the pelvis or an anorectal ultrasound may be recommended by your physician.

### What over-the-counter treatments or home remedies can be used for perianal Crohn's disease?

A high-fiber diet, sitz baths, and local anesthetic creams may be helpful.

### What prescription medications are used for perianal Crohn's disease and how do they work?

Anti-inflammatory agents can be helpful in decreasing the inflammation associated with perianal Crohn's disease. Antibiotics, especially metronidazole (Flagyl), appear to remove some of the bacteria that can fuel and worsen this condition. Immunomodulating agents such as 6-mercaptopurine and azathioprine may be helpful as well. These agents reduce the inflammation associated with Crohn's disease that triggers the development of perianal problems. Infliximab (Remicade), an intravenously administered anti-inflammatory agent, is also effective for healing perianal fistulas.

### What nonsurgical procedures can be used to treat perianal Crohn's disease?

Anal strictures can be stretched in the clinic or operating room.

### Is surgery ever used as a treatment for perianal Crohn's disease?

Yes. Approximately 4% of patients with Crohn's disease will eventually need surgery for perianal complications.

### When is surgery used to treat perianal Crohn's disease?

Surgical drainage is used to treat perianal abscesses. Surgery is also used for symptomatic draining of fistulas or painful fissures that do not improve with medical treatment. The primary goal for surgery for perianal Crohn's disease is to improve quality of life and alleviate discomfort.

### Which surgical procedures are performed for the treatment of perianal Crohn's disease?

Drainage of abscesses, placement of drains or setons (a piece of fabric, gauze, or wire used to keep a sinus track open while it heals) in symptomatic fistulas, fistulotomy (removal of the fistula), and stretching of the anal strictures. Sometimes an artificial flap needs to be placed to assist with wound healing after removal of the fistula. In some patients, an ileostomy with or without removal of the rectum is required.

## What additional information should I know about perianal Crohn's disease?

The management of perianal Crohn's disease often requires the combined efforts of a medical and surgical specialist.

# Chapter 8.7

# Pruritus ani

## What is pruritus ani?

Pruritus ani is the term used to describe itching of the tissue and skin of the anal and groin areas.

## How does pruritus ani occur?

There is usually no complete explanation as to why patients develop pruritus ani. The majority of cases happen because patients irritate the anal region through excessive rubbing and exposure to soaps and perfumes. Some patients with pruritus ani may have a small amount of leakage of the rectal contents, which adds to the irritation of the area.

## What are the symptoms of pruritus ani?

Itchiness of the anal area and groin. Sometimes severe skin irritation, damage, and abnormal healing of the perianal skin may cause bleeding and pain around the anus and groin.

## Are there any other conditions that cause the same symptoms as pruritus ani?

A variety of conditions can cause anal itching. These include skin conditions such as eczema and psoriasis, infection with pinworms and yeasts, systemic diseases such as diabetes, psychogenic disorders such as anxiety, and dietary factors including smoking and consumption of coffee, milk, tomatoes, chocolate, nuts, citrus fruits, and alcoholic beverages.

## What factors increase the risk of developing pruritus ani?

Excessive rubbing and cleansing of the anal region with soaps and perfumes that irritate the skin. The condition may worsen with further exposure of the affected area to strong cleansing agents such as alkaline soaps, alcohol, and witch hazel.

## Can pruritus ani predispose to cancer?

No. However, anal cancers may cause pruritus ani.

### What tests are performed to diagnose pruritus ani?

A detailed examination of the anus and skin surrounding the anus and groin may reveal changes suggestive of the diagnosis. Additionally, this examination may help to diagnose other conditions that cause anal itching. A scraping or biopsy of the affected area is sometimes helpful to rule out infections and chronic skin diseases. An anoscopy or sigmoidoscopy to look at the anus and rectum may be required. Sometimes a full colonoscopy may be recommended.

### What over-the-counter treatments or home remedies can be used for pruritus ani?

Dietary management with elimination of the foods mentioned above may be helpful. Adding fiber supplements and increasing dietary fiber is often beneficial. Cleansing the anal region after going to the bathroom with warm water and/or cleansing towelettes (which do not contain alcohol or witch hazel) is recommended. Colloidal oatmeal baths may also help. Talcum powder has been recommended as being beneficial. Moisturizing and lubricating skin ointments such as Balneol and Tucks are helpful. A cotton ball may be placed near the anus to absorb excessive rectal discharge.

### What prescription medications are used for pruritus ani and how do they work?

Some ointments containing hydrocortisone such as Analpram HC or Proctocream may be used on a limited basis. These agents decrease inflammation of the damaged perianal skin.

### What nonsurgical procedures can be used to treat pruritus ani?

Biofeedback therapy (a form of pelvic muscle retraining) and hypnosis have been shown to help in some patients.

### Is surgery ever used as a treatment for pruritus ani?

No.

### What additional information should I know about pruritus ani?

This condition is more common in men than women. Most physicians agree that patients with pruritus ani benefit greatly from understanding the factors that worsen the condition.

# Chapter 8.8

# Radiation proctopathy

*(also known as: radiation proctitis)*

### What is radiation proctopathy?

Radiation proctopathy is the damage to the rectum and/or anus that occurs in patients who are undergoing or have previously received radiation therapy to the pelvic organs, including the prostate, uterus, and ovaries.

### How does radiation proctopathy occur?

Because the rectum is next to the prostate in men, and the uterus and ovaries in women, rectal injury may occur from radiation treatment for cancer of these organs.

### What are the symptoms of radiation proctopathy?

During radiation therapy, diarrhea and the urge to move the bowels may occur. From 6 months to many years after completion of radiation therapy, some patients may experience rectal bleeding, diarrhea, urge to move the bowels without actually having a bowel movement, difficulty passing stool, and fecal incontinence.

### Are there any other conditions that cause the same symptoms as radiation proctopathy?

Rectal or anal cancer, ulcerative proctitis or colitis, rectocele, and irritable bowel syndrome.

### What factors increase the risk of developing radiation proctopathy?

Radiation treatment for pelvic cancer.

### Can radiation proctopathy predispose to cancer?

Rarely. However, another cancer may form at the site of prior radiation treatment.

### What tests are performed to diagnose radiation proctopathy?

Flexible sigmoidoscopy, or colonoscopy if rectal bleeding is present.

### What over-the-counter treatments or home remedies can be used for radiation proctopathy?

If symptoms occur during radiation therapy, a low fiber diet, loperamide (Imodium), and/or kaolin and pectin (Kaopectate) are used to relieve diarrhea. For symptoms that occur 6 months after completion of therapy, vitamins A, C, and E may be helpful.

### What prescription medications are used for radiation proctopathy and how do they work?

Sucralfate (Carafate) may decrease bleeding by protecting the surface of the rectum. Estrogens with progesterone may decrease bleeding; however, the mechanism of action is unknown. Corticosteroids (prednisone) and 5-ASA (aspirin) compounds (Asacol, Azulfidine, Dipentum) may reduce associated inflammation.

### What nonsurgical procedures can be used to treat radiation proctopathy?

For bleeding, the following nonsurgical procedures are used: endoscopy with application of electrocautery or argon plasma coagulation; application of formaldehyde to bleeding areas; hyperbaric oxygen treatment.

### Is surgery ever used as a treatment for radiation proctopathy?

Yes.

### When is surgery used to treat radiation proctopathy?

When bleeding cannot be stopped or when the condition is complicated by extreme narrowing of the bowel, obstruction of the bowel, or abnormal connection (fistula) of the bowel to other organs such as the bladder or vagina.

### What surgical procedures are performed for the treatment of radiation proctopathy?

Creation of a colostomy (a connection between the bowel and the abdominal wall that drains feces through a bag) to divert stool away from the rectum. In some carefully selected patients with large ulcers, blockages, or bleeding that will not stop, the rectum is removed (a proctectomy). In its place, a new rectum may be constructed from the remaining colon, which is connected to the anus (this surgery is called a colonic J pouch construction).

### What additional information should I know about radiation proctopathy?

This condition is sometimes confused with ulcerative proctitis or colitis. Unlike these conditions, there is little inflammation associated with radiation proctopathy. Radiation proctopathy is likely to become more common as radiation therapy is used more often as a first-line treatment for pelvic cancer.

# Chapter 8.9

# Rectal prolapse

## What is a rectal prolapse?

A rectal prolapse is a condition in which a portion of the lining of the rectum or the entire rectal wall protrudes into, and at times outside of, the anus.

## How does rectal prolapse occur?

Most patients begin with symptoms of constipation and straining. The lining of the rectal tissue becomes loose and begins to protrude toward the anus. Often, the colon is also elongated and floppy, causing worse constipation and straining. Frequent straining appears to exacerbate the condition because it damages the nerves that supply the rectum and anus. This allows for further loosening of the anal sphincter and easier passage of rectal tissue through the anal canal.

## What are the symptoms of rectal prolapse?

Persons with rectal prolapse will notice a protrusion at the anus or outside of the anus when going to the bathroom, or straining when attempting to pass a stool. Bleeding, anal itching, and anal and rectal pain are also common symptoms. Patients may have to push the protruding rectal tissue back up into the anus. Severe pain and fever suggest that the blood supply to the prolapsed rectum is being compromised and may constitute a medical emergency.

## Are there any other conditions that cause the same symptoms as rectal prolapse?

Prolapsed hemorrhoids, anal fissure, anal sphincter dysfunction, other forms of constipation, and solitary rectal ulcer syndrome all cause similar symptoms.

## What factors increase the risk of developing rectal prolapse?

A history of straining or constipation is an important factor. Other diseases that are associated with rectal prolapse include spinal cord disorders, cystic fibrosis, congenital neurologic diseases, Marfan's syndrome, and schistosomiasis. It is estimated that up to 5% of patients with rectal prolapse have a rectal or sigmoid colon cancer, therefore, it is important to be tested for these if you have this condition.

## Can rectal prolapse predispose to cancer?

No. However, rectal prolapse may be secondary to a cancer of the colon or rectum.

### What tests are performed to diagnose rectal prolapse?

The diagnosis of rectal prolapse is generally made with a physical examination. Other tests may include dynamic proctography to document the presence of prolapse. A flexible sigmoidoscopy or colonoscopy is performed to rule out a rectal or sigmoid colon cancer. Anorectal manometry or pudendal nerve terminal latency measurements may be performed to test for other abnormalities of the anorectal region.

### What over-the-counter treatments or home remedies can be used for rectal prolapse?

For milder cases, fiber supplementation, sitz baths, and local anesthetic creams may be beneficial.

### What prescription medications are used for rectal prolapse?

None.

### What nonsurgical procedures can be used to treat rectal prolapse?

None.

### Is surgery ever used as a treatment for rectal prolapse?

Yes, surgery is used in almost all cases of rectal prolapse.

### When is surgery used to treat rectal prolapse?

If rectal prolapse is associated with fecal incontinence, severe constipation, rectal bleeding, or a prolapse of the entire rectal wall. Surgery is only avoided in minor cases of prolapse in which the lining of the rectum does not extend past the anus. This condition is called rectoanal intussusception.

### What surgical procedures are performed for the treatment of rectal prolapse?

Excess rectal tissue is removed. The remaining rectum is attached to the pelvic bones to hold it in place and prevent further prolapse.

### What additional information should I know about rectal prolapse?

This condition is up to 10-times more common in women than in men. It generally occurs after the age of 50 years.

# Chapter 8.10

# Solitary rectal ulcer syndrome

### What is solitary rectal ulcer syndrome?

Solitary rectal ulcer syndrome (SRUS) is a rare, chronic condition characterized by inflammation and ulceration of a portion of the lining of the rectum, often seen in patients suffering from chronic constipation.

### How does SRUS develop?

This condition develops when there is decreased blood flow to the lining of the rectum. It appears to occur when portions of the lining of the rectum move towards and sometimes outside of the anus (rectal prolapse), or when intense anal spasm occurs when attempting to defecate.

### What are the symptoms of SRUS?

The most common symptom of SRUS is rectal bleeding. Other symptoms include constipation, rectal pain, passage of mucus in the stool, and back or hip pain.

### Are there any other conditions that cause the same symptoms as SRUS?

Ulcerative proctitis, Crohn's disease, rectal and anal cancers, hemorrhoids, and conditions that cause constipation such as nonrelaxing puborectalis syndrome.

### What factors increase the risk of developing SRUS?

Constipation, straining, rectal prolapse, removal of stool from the rectum with a finger, and anal sexual activity.

### Can SRUS predispose to cancer?

No.

### What tests are performed to diagnose SRUS?

A physical examination of the anus and rectum is required to check for rectal prolapse. Flexible sigmoidoscopy and colonoscopy are used to visualize the affected area of the rectum. Biopsies may be performed to rule out other sources of rectal bleeding.

### What over-the-counter treatments or home remedies can be used for SRUS?

Avoidance of straining on the toilet. Stool softeners such as Colace (dioctyl sodium sulfosuccinate); bulking agents such as psyllium (Metamucil, Konsyl), methylcellulose (Citrucel), or calcium polycarbophyl (FiberCon, Konsyl); or other laxatives such as milk of magnesia or mineral oil. Enemas may also assist with stool passage.

### What prescription medications are used for SRUS and how do they work?

Hydrocortisone enemas may be effective by reducing the inflammation of the rectal lining. Sucralfate enemas may assist in healing the affected area.

### What nonsurgical procedures can be used to treat SRUS?

Botulinum toxin (Botox) injections into the anal sphincter may be used if the anal sphincter is tight (but not for patients with a rectal prolapse). Botox relaxes the sphincter and allows for better evacuation of feces and avoidance of straining.

### Is surgery ever used as a treatment for SRUS?

Yes.

### When is surgery used to treat SRUS?

When symptoms persist despite lifestyle modifications and medical therapy.

### What surgical procedures are performed for the treatment of SRUS?

If rectal prolapse causes the SRUS, a rectopexy or strengthening of the lining of the rectum can be performed. If spasm of the anus is causing this condition, the puborectalis muscle may be cut.

### What additional information should I know about SRUS?

This is a relatively uncommon condition. The diagnosis of SRUS may be difficult. Some patients with this condition may be diagnosed as having Crohn's disease, ulcerative colitis, or rectal masses or cancers. Careful medical history, sigmoidoscopy or colonoscopy, and biopsies of the affected area all assist greatly in confirming this diagnosis.

# Chapter 8.11

# Ulcerative proctitis

## What is ulcerative proctitis?

Ulcerative proctitis is a chronic inflammatory disease of the rectum.

## How does ulcerative proctitis occur?

Ulcerative proctitis is an autoimmune disorder characterized by antibodies that attack the inside lining of the rectum. The inflammation probably occurs in people who have a genetic predisposition to develop the disease. When these individuals are exposed to a protein (probably from a bacteria or other substance inside the rectum), chemicals are secreted that stimulate the immune system to produce rectal inflammation.

## What are the symptoms of ulcerative proctitis?

Diarrhea and rectal bleeding are the most common symptoms. An urgency to move the bowels, rectal pain, fecal incontinence, and a sense of incomplete evacuation may also occur. Some patients with more severe disease develop fever, weight loss, and a low blood count.

## Are there any other conditions that cause the same symptoms as ulcerative proctitis?

Colitis involving other portions of the colon can cause similar symptoms. Crohn's disease may also cause similar symptoms. Diarrhea may be due to infection and rectal bleeding can occur due to colonic or rectal polyps, colonic or rectal cancer, hemorrhoids, diverticulosis, and medications such as aspirin or ibuprofen.

## What factors increase the risk of developing ulcerative proctitis?

A family history of ulcerative colitis or Crohn's disease.

## Can ulcerative proctitis predispose to cancer?

Yes. However, cancer is rare from ulcerative proctitis alone and is more common when ulcerative colitis is present and involves the entire colon.

## What tests are performed to diagnose ulcerative proctitis?

Flexible sigmoidoscopy. Colonoscopy is also used to determine the extent of colonic involvement and later for surveillance.

### What over-the-counter treatments or home remedies can be used for ulcerative proctitis?

Fiber therapy may be beneficial in some patients in alleviating symptoms such as urgency.

### What prescription medicines are used for ulcerative proctitis and how do they work?

Mild to moderate disease is treated initially with 5-ASA (5-aminosalicylic acid [aspirin]) containing agents administered either orally or rectally. Mesalamine suppositories are recommended. These medications work directly on the lining of the rectum to stop the inflammation. More severe disease is treated with prednisone. Prednisone suppresses the immune system and stops the inflammation. Patients who have chronic, ongoing symptoms are treated with the immunomodulating agents 6-mercaptopurine or azathioprine. These cause long-term suppression of the inflammation.

### What nonsurgical procedures can be used to treat ulcerative proctitis?

None.

### Is surgery ever used as a treatment for ulcerative proctitis?

Yes.

### When is surgery used to treat ulcerative proctitis?

When symptoms cannot be controlled with medication; or, if colon cancer develops in affected areas of the colon or changes are occurring in the colonic tissues that predispose to the development of cancer.

### What surgical procedures are performed for the treatment of ulcerative proctitis?

In the past, a colectomy (removal of the colon) and ileostomy (the small intestine is attached to the abdominal wall and a bag outside of the body) were used to surgically treat ulcerative proctitis (and ulcerative colitis). Now, removal of the colon (proctocolectomy) and creation of a new colon from a portion of the small intestine (ileoanal pouch anastomosis or J pouch) is the surgical treatment of choice for ulcerative proctitis (and ulcerative colitis).

### What additional information should I know about ulcerative proctitis?

You should have a full colonoscopy with biopsies throughout the colon for surveillance every 2–3 years after symptoms of ulcerative proctitis have been present for 10 years or more.

# Chapter 8.12

# Venereal warts

*(also known as: condylomata acuminata)*

## What are venereal warts?

Venereal warts are skin abnormalities characterized by pink/gray swellings near the anal region and sometimes extending to the genital area. They are often described as having a cauliflower-like appearance.

## How do venereal warts occur?

They are caused by a viral infection from the human papilloma virus. This infection is sexually transmitted and is highly contagious.

## What are the symptoms of venereal warts?

The most common symptoms of venereal warts are a sense of fullness around the anal or genital region, itching, pain, bleeding from the affected area, and rectal, vaginal, or penile discharge.

## Are there any other conditions that cause the same symptoms as venereal warts?

Pruritus ani and skin conditions involving the anal or genital area.

## What factors increase the risk of developing venereal warts?

Sexual activity with individuals who have venereal warts or are infected with the virus that causes this condition predisposes to the development of venereal warts. Persons who are sexually promiscuous, homosexual males with other sexually transmitted diseases, HIV-infected individuals, and victims of sexual abuse due to spread of the infection from the abuser to their victim.

## Can venereal warts predispose to cancer?

Yes. Venereal warts are a risk factor for the development of squamous cell carcinoma of the anorectal region and carcinoma of the cervix and of other portions of the genital tract.

### What tests are performed to diagnose venereal warts?

The diagnosis is usually made by a physical examination of the affected area. Sometimes biopsies are obtained. A proctoscopy or flexible sigmoidoscopy may be required to determine whether there are additional warts present in the anus or rectum that cannot be visualized externally.

### What over-the-counter treatments or home remedies can be used for venereal warts?

None.

### What prescription medications are used for venereal warts and how do they work?

Podofilox (Condylox) may be prescribed by your physician. It is a topical destructive agent that you apply directly to the warts. It works by stopping the cells in the warts from multiplying. Imiquimod (Aldara) is another topical destructive cream that is applied to the warts. It appears to destroy the warts by causing secretion of chemicals called cytokines, which stimulate an inflammatory reaction that is used to fight off the infection. Podophyllum is also a topical destructive agent, but it has to be applied by your physician. It destroys the tissue containing the warts.

### What nonsurgical procedures can be used to treat venereal warts?

Laser therapy is often successful. Burning of the warts with electrocautery is also highly successful. Your physician may also consider injecting the warts with medications that cause their destruction including chemotherapy drugs and Interferon. Cryotherapy, which involves applying liquid nitrogen to the warts, is also used.

### Is surgery ever used as a treatment for venereal warts?

Yes.

### When is surgery used to treat venereal warts?

Surgery is used for large warts that cannot be successfully removed with other therapies. Surgery may also be used for warts that keep coming back, and warts that are in the anal canal and rectum.

### What surgical procedures are performed for the treatment of venereal warts?

The warts and a portion of the surrounding normal skin are surgically removed. This is usually performed in conjunction with burning of the affected area using electrocautery.

### What additional information should I know about venereal warts?

Since venereal warts are considered to be a risk factor for cancers of the anal and genital regions, periodic examinations of the affected areas are necessary. Women with venereal warts should undergo frequent Pap smears and genital examinations.

# Abbreviations

| | |
|---|---|
| 5-ASA | 5-aminosalicylic acid |
| 5-FU | 5-fluorouracil |
| 5-HIAA | 5-hydroxyindole acetic acid |
| *APC* | adenomatous polyposis coli |
| APR | abdominoperineal resection |
| Cl | chloride |
| CT | computed tomography |
| DALM | dysplasia-associated lesion or mass |
| *DCC* | deleted in colon cancer |
| EAS | external anal sphincter |
| EMG | electromyography |
| FAP | familial adenomatous polyposis |
| $HCO_3$ | bicarbonate |
| HPV | human papillomavirus |
| HPZ | high-pressure zone |
| HSV-2 | herpes simplex virus 2 |
| IAS | internal anal sphincter |
| IV | intravenous |
| IVBP | intravenous piggyback |
| K | potassium |
| LGV | lymphogranuloma venereum |
| MEN | multiple endocrine neoplasia |
| Mg | magnesium |
| MRI | magnetic resonance imaging |
| Na | sodium |
| NHANES | National Health and Nutrition Examination Survey |
| NHIS | National Health Interview Survey |
| PNTML | pudendal nerve terminal motor latency |
| RAIR | rectoanal inhibitory reflex |
| SRUS | solitary rectal ulcer syndrome |
| TNM | tumor, nodes, metastases |

# Further reading

## Textbooks


Barnes L, Corman ML, editors. *Colon and Rectal Surgery*. 4th ed. Philadelphia, PA: Lippincott–Raven Publishers, 1998.

Feldman M, Friedman LS, Sleisenger MH, editors. *Sleisenger & Fordtran's Gastrointestinal and Liver Disease*. 7th ed. Philadelphia, PA: Saunders, 2002.

Yamada T, editor. *Textbook of Gastroenterology*. 2nd ed. Philadelphia, PA: Lippincott Williams & Wilkins, 1995.

Gordon PH, Nivatvongs S, editors. *Principles and Practice of Surgery for the Colon, Rectum and Anus*. 2nd ed. New York, NY: Marcel Dekker, 1999.

Gorbach SL, Bartlett JG, Blacklow NR, editors. *Infectious Diseases*. 2nd ed. Philadelphia, PA: Saunders, 1997.


## Review articles


Wald A. Anorectal and pelvic pain in women: diagnostic considerations and treatment. *J Clin Gastroenterol.* 2001;33(4):283–8.

Nelson R. Anorectal abscess fistula: what do we know? *Surg Clin North Am.* 2002;82(6):1139–51.

Bartram C. Dynamic evaluation of the anorectum. *Radiol Clin North Am.* 2003;41(2):425–41.

Bharucha AE. Fecal incontinence. *Gastroenterology.* 2003;124(6):1672–85.

Gopal DV. Diseases of the rectum and anus: a clinical approach to common disorders. *Clin Cornerstone.* 2002;4(4):34–48.

Utzig MJ, Kroesen AJ, Buhr HJ. Concepts in pathogenesis and treatment of chronic anal fissure – a review of the literature. *Am J Gastroenterol.* 2003;98(5):968–74.

Hong JJ, Park W, Ehrenpreis ED. Review article: current therapeutic options for radiation proctopathy. *Aliment Pharmacol Ther.* 2001;15(9):1253–62.

Maria G, Sganga G, Civello IM, Brisinda G. Botulinum neurotoxin and other treatments for fissure-in-ano and pelvic floor disorders. *B J Surg.* 2002;89(8):950–61.

Olsen AL, Rao SS. Clinical neurophysiology and electrodiagnostic testing of the pelvic floor. *Gastroenterol Clin North Am.* 2001;30(1):33–54,v–vi.

Moore HG, Guillem JG. Anal neoplasms. *Surg Clin North Am.* 2002;82(6):1233–51.

Moore HG, Guillem JG. Multimodality management of locally advanced rectal cancer. *Am Surg.* 2003;69(7):612–9.

Schmitt SL, Wexner SD. Treatment of anorectal manifestations of AIDS. *Int J STD AIDS.* 1994;5(1):8–10.

# Index